The Support Group Sourcebook

What They Are,
How You Can Find One,
and How They Can Help You

L I N D A L . K L E I N

JOHN WILEY & SONS, INC.

New York • Chichester • Weinheim • Brisbane • Singapore • Toronto

Published by John Wiley & Sons, Inc.
Published simultaneously in Canada.

This publication is designed to provide accurate and authoritative information in regard to the subject matter covered. It is sold with the understanding that the publisher is not engaged in rendering professional services. If professional advice or other expert assistance is required, the services of a competent professional person should be sought.

Library of Congress Cataloging in Publication Data

Klein, Linda
    The support group sourcebook: what they are, how you can find one, and how they can help you / Linda L. Klein.
        p. cm.
    Includes index.
    ISBN 0-471-34789-2 (paper)
    1. Self-help groups. 2. Social interaction. 3. Intergroup relations.
I. Title.

HV547 .K58 2000
361.4—dc21

99-049351

Printed in the United States of America

10 9 8 7 6 5 4 3 2 1

This book is dedicated to

The people I love the most
My husband Bill
My daughter Mary
My son Andrew
My daughter Alison
My mother Esther

The person who loved me the most
My mother
Esther Gustafson Wick
B. June 2, 1907–D. January 9, 1997

The person who loved my mother the most
The Grandmother I never knew
The reason for the work I do
Hilda Josephine Gustafson
B. October 21, 1873–D. October 27, 1918

Contents

Acknowledgments

A book about the value of support groups is truly the collective wisdom of all the individuals who have participated in groups or have been involved in group leadership. In my work in support groups, I have come in contact with many kindred souls, including:

Jane Klein, college roommate and thirty-plus-year soulmate. Jane introduced me to the magic of support groups. We have been blessed by a long, rewarding relationship—both personally and professionally.

Sue Harvieux, the facilitator of the first support group I ever attended. Sue taught me that volunteering your time with compassion, empathy, and caring are far more important than having a full-time job.

Sister Ann Michele Jadlowski, CSJ, long-time hospital chaplain and support group leader, at HealthEast St. Joseph's Hospital. Sister Ann, one of my favorite nuns, taught me the value of being truly present for people who are suffering.

Nancy Salscheider, support group leader extraordinaire and one of the most valuable patient advocates ever created. Nancy taught me the importance of having a sense of humor and just "being yourself." Because she is so caring and accessible, her voice mail is always full and she never stops working.

Donna Hemer, true friend and fellow support group leader. Our friendship is an example of the rich benefits to be derived from developing a group of kindred souls.

Dennis, Kate, Joan, Sister Arne, Jackie, Randy and Sheri, Ed and Marge, Pat, Lea, Gwen, and any other specific support group members whose experiences were shared in this book.

In addition to these specific individuals, I want to thank all the members of Nancy and my Finding Your Way support group, one of the "coolest groups" on the planet; all the members of Donna and my Affirming Life support group, some of the most honest and endearing women in the world; and to Nancy Grandt and the members of the breast cancer support group that I cofacilitated for several years.

I also want to thank the people at the National Stroke Association for inviting me and my coauthor Judi Johnson to develop *Discovery Circles,* a manual for stroke support group leaders. The research and writing of that manual served as a valuable guide for this book. I am also indebted to the Leukemia Society of America (LSA) for providing ongoing support and training for support group facilitators across the country.

I am proud that during the time this book was being written, my original publisher Chronimed was acquired by John Wiley & Sons, Inc. Because of that, I had the assistance of a wonderful editor, Betsy Thorpe, who helped me to sort out the nuts and bolts of group leadership from the intuitive insights and experiences of the group members.

I want to thank Rachel Naomi Remen, M.D., for writing *Kitchen Table Wisdom,* which constantly reminds me that the depth of human relationships and connections is truly all that really matters in life.

Finally, thank you in advance to every person who reads this book and takes it upon him or herself to either start or become involved in a support group. You have done yourself a favor.

Preface
Why This Book?
A Personal Glimpse

THE LEGACY

Every morning when my youngest child gets on the school bus, I make it a point to examine every little thing about her—the curl of her hair, the soft freckles borne of biking in the sun, the hazel eyes that captivated me from the moment she was born. Sometimes she leans over just so slightly to be hugged, and I am honored. She's 12 now, almost a teenager. Those signs of affection will soon fade.

When my own mother, Esther, was 12, my grandmother died of ovarian cancer. She was just 45. My mother, the fifth in a family of eight children, had been a favored child. When she was afflicted with head lice and forced to shave her head, my grandmother insisted that mother's younger sister Evelyn also shave her head—so Esther wouldn't look so obvious. Mother had been a much-loved child. After her mother's death, she developed a reverence for motherhood. As a result, the six children in my family were loved unconditionally—as she had been loved.

Because of this history, I became paranoid over the word cancer *at a very young age. When I would see the seven danger signals printed on the back of a cereal box or in a magazine, I would quickly turn the page. I believed that if I read those danger signals, I was certain to recognize at least one telltale symptom—either in myself or in my mother. I loved my mother deeply and could not imagine being without her.*

When my baby turns 13, it will be a milestone for me. That birthday will verify that we have survived the family legacy. But my deep love for her—and for my other children—has taught me another valuable lesson. When I was younger, I had only considered the child's view—the fear and the devastation that a 12-year-old would feel on losing her mother. I hadn't considered how equally devastating it must have been for my grandmother to finally accept that she was leaving all those beautiful children behind. Her baby Everett was only two. Photographs of her still haunt me with all the "what might have beens" that they provoke.

The legacy of this story is my involvement in cancer care. At some point, I knew that I would spend the rest of my life finding ways to ease the pain, both for individuals living with cancer and for the loved ones they might potentially leave behind.

Because I grew up fearing cancer, as an adult I decided to conquer my fear by learning more about it. I went to Judi Johnson, who had developed the American Cancer Society's I Can Cope patient-education program, and told her I was interested in writing a book about the program. She agreed to collaborate. While researching and writing that book, *I Can Cope: Staying Healthy with Cancer,* I spent many hours in class getting to know people recently diagnosed with cancer. During each class series, I watched a miraculous process. The first night, we started with a room full of strangers. By the end of the last class, those strangers had become friends. Most had gone from being fearful to being courageous. Not only had they learned about cancer, they had learned how to live with cancer. By graduation night, these people could once again laugh and enjoy themselves. From this whole experience, I learned that the support of like-minded individuals has an immensely positive effect on recovery and healing.

Once the book was completed, I enrolled in training to become a group leader. For the past 10 years, I have been a volunteer facilitator for a variety of groups. Although the groups meet for different reasons, the group dynamic is almost always the same—people helping people. The group members come together as strangers and evolve into kindred souls. Regardless of their life experience—whether it be chronic illness, chemical dependency, abuse, depression, death and grieving, or alternative lifestyles—kindred souls learn one very important lesson: *They are not alone.* They come to experience what Cornelius Ryan called "the bond that surpasses a healthy person's understanding."

ABOUT THE BOOK

This book came about for two reasons. First, I wanted the general public to know that support groups involve much more than simply setting up a circle of folding chairs in a meeting room and letting people take turns complaining about things. Yet I knew when I started writing the book that it would be difficult to put the magic of support group into words. After all, it is not a one-dimensional experience. Things happen among people in that room that can only be felt with the heart. That's why I tried to tell much of the story by introducing you to some of the group members. By seeing the experience through the members' eyes, perhaps you can better understand exactly what happened to them. And, just by chance, you might then begin to wonder if the same thing could happen to you. (Believe me, it can!)

Second, I wanted to help those of you who would really like to start a group and don't quite know how to proceed. Certainly, you don't need a college course to get a group going. But there are some strategies that can help—especially in the formative stages. In every section of this book, you will be hearing the perspectives of both the group leader and the group members. Keep in mind that, for the most part, each individual in the group will be a greater asset to the group process if she or he is skilled enough to play either role. For instance, learning how to listen well and how to ask probing questions are important skills for both the group leader *and* the group members. If all group members understand the key ingredients of successful groups, they can make a conscious effort to inject those ingredients into the group. On the other hand, they can consciously look for and avoid the bad habits that sometimes doom groups to eventual failure.

At the end of several chapters are Discussion Guides. The key word here is *discussion*. (One of the easiest traps for maturing groups to fall into is the temptation to just chat.) These guides are provided as a means to take your group sharing to a higher level—if that is the direction you wish to go. Please remember that this type of discussion can be initiated by any group member—it is not necessarily the responsibility of the group leader. In fact, if everyone in the group read the discussion guide prior to the meeting, everyone would arrive prepared for the topical discussion.

The last chapter of the book, P.S. So You Want to Be a Group Leader, is devoted to giving specific direction to group leaders, including possible press releases or public service announcements (PSAs). Feel free to take at least a peek at this section, however, even if beginning a group is not your intention. Many of the pointers can also help group members learn how to be better participants. And the information just might be the extra nudge you need to start your own group—which leads me to the most important reason of all for writing this book.

I hope many people read this book, of course, including all the people who are already members of some type of support group. But most important, I hope the cynics and the skeptics and the loners are reading this book—the people who say "I'm coping just fine" when I suggest attending I Can Cope classes—because, deep in our hearts, none of us is *really* coping just fine, no matter what our life situation. Rather, we often feel lonely and fearful. In a complex and highly technical world, we continue to search for meaningful connections. At three o'clock in the morning, when we are wide awake and staring at the ceiling, we wonder deep inside if we are the only ones who feel this way—so alone.

A community of kindred souls affirms for us that we are not alone. To find that community, you may need to shed your cynicism and skepticism. You may need to swallow your pride and admit that people *do* need people in order to be fully human. I hope this book emboldens and encourages you to start the process: to pick up the phone and make an inquiry, to type up a notice and post it on a bulletin board, to search the Internet for a connection that works. Because for the past 10 years, in all my associations with support groups, I have felt the magic in every one. All those kindred souls couldn't be wrong.

Introduction
Searching for Community in an Internet World

Without friends, no one would choose to live, even if he had all other goods.

—ARISTOTLE

In his leisure time, my husband, Bill, is a woodcutter. Thanks to his efforts, we have been heating our 100-year-old home with wood since moving to this hobby farm 11 years ago. About five years ago, his boss at AT&T bought a large piece of wooded land not far from our home. As he developed the land, cutting it into nine small lots, he asked Bill to help clear some of the trees to make way for "executive homesites."

Since that time, Bill has spent many weekend hours on that land and has gotten to know the new landowners on a first-name basis—one is an executive at 3M. Another is a retired anesthesiologist with two black labradors—Bill calls him "Doc." Another is a land developer with young children. Recently, Bill was asked to remove some victims of oak wilt from the homesite of a middle-aged couple—the husband is a physician (a pediatric specialist), and the wife owns a small interior design business. They have three grown sons. The home, with its "all-white" interior, isn't suited to real woodburning—just no-mess gas logs. So they are happy to have Bill spend time clearing out the dead trees. Last weekend, he casually asked Mrs. a question about one of the neighbors. She gave him an odd look and replied: "Oh, we haven't met any of the neighbors."

Contrast this response with what would have been more likely in the neighborhoods in which many of us grew up. My family lived next door to the Koppens; and from diapers to grade school to graduation, we grew up with the Koppen children. For years, tall, stately Betty Koppen sat at our kitchen table with a cup of coffee and a cigarette. Her visits sometimes stretched from morning into afternoon. Other days, my mother went to Betty's house. Once a week, they got together a foursome for bridge. Through it all, they knew one another's ups and downs, pleasures and pains.

When Betty was diagnosed with breast cancer at the young age of 36, the world wasn't ready to talk about cancer yet—not in polite company. Her husband Bob, a hard-working, highway-department employee, retreated to the solace of his beloved vegetable garden. Her children didn't know what was happening. But my mother did. Betty's visits to our kitchen table became more frequent. She stayed longer—and she got thinner. Finally, one day the ambulance came to taken Betty's slight body away. In the beginning, my mother and Betty might not have chosen one another as friends. But they became kindred souls just the same. And they were better off for it.

We scheme about the future,
And we dream about the past,
When just a simple reaching out
Might build a bridge that lasts.

—JOHN HIATT

The United States evolved as a nation of individualists, proud of their independence, uncommitted to anyone but themselves. Yet over the years, the social fabric woven by that rugged individualism has begun to unfurl. Families are separated by distance and by lack of time. Thanks to advanced electronic communication, we speak through the Internet and voice mail, diminishing our face-to-face contact with one another. Paradoxically, in the midst of this high-tech, instant-communication global society, many Americans live in isolation—anonymous lives lived out on executive homesites.

As it turns out, realizing the American dream of acquiring wealth and power has not brought with it the expected happiness and self-satisfaction. We own our own homes—many of them starter castles—but our doors are figuratively and literally closed and locked to keep out strangers. Small-town communities and small social and religious organizations are dying out. More and more people are facing life on their own—just at a time when perhaps they need other people most. Who will watch out for us in times of trouble? If we move so often that the direct-mail firms are unable to maintain current lists, where will we develop emotionally supportive friendships?

From our early fierce independence, we have now evolved into a nation of "people needing people," in search of a way to escape our self-inflicted isolation and to reconnect with others in a safe, intimate environment.

In and through community lies the salvation of the world.

—M. Scott Peck

People who need people seek the comfort of community. They want to feel safe among others, to know that they (and their opinions) are valued, and to feel a sense of connection to one another on a very personal level. But in today's society, we are no longer born into community. Now, in many cases, we must *choose* our community. To accomplish a renewed sense of togetherness, groups of like-minded individuals are starting to create new communities in which kindred souls can find predictable and rewarding human contact in an unpredictable world. They gather together to be encouraged, supported, and loved. The members of one Native American tribe call their fellow group members "shoulder friends." These new communities reinforce a law of quantum physics—*the nature of reality is a dynamic relationship, not isolated units of matter.* And because U.S. society is mobile and fluid, individuals may end up forming these new communities again and again—in new locations and for the specific purposes of many different affinity groups.

Unlike past communities (neighborhoods and families), these new intentional groups focus on the individual's higher level of emotional and spiritual needs, as opposed to physical or monetary needs. Through discussion, storytelling, and sharing the emotions involved in everyday life, group members help each other to understand their own identity. In a rapidly changing world, it is comforting to share the "journey into an unknown future" with a group of kindred souls.

When the requirements of a true community are met—*personal commitment, vulnerability,* and *honesty*—the group commitment draws individuals out of themselves, yanks them from their isolated lives, and gently places them in a safe environment where they can share their needs, feel understood and accepted, gain courage, and experience inner healing.

This book is about people who joined groups and what happened to them through the group process. It is about pain and loss, illness and addiction, grief and death. Through it all, the people you will meet continue to find value and meaning in their lives. Their groups have helped them reach that point.

This book is also about leading groups. It is about the process of natural group evolution, with specific guidelines to give you confidence if you are a group leader.

Whether you lead a group, join a group, or are just curious about the process, this book should remind you of the importance of staying connected to others.

Many of us under fifty years old have never known the feeling of a small town, the camaraderie around a "potbelly stove" or even friends and neighbors we can know and trust.

—BILL KAUTH

FOUR LIVES IN CRISIS

Donna

At the age of 47, Donna was on top of the world. Both of her sons had recently graduated from college; her husband's law practice was thriving; she had completed her master's degree and was enjoying her career as a psychologist. Then a routine mammogram turned her world upside down. The diagnosis: a fast-growing breast cancer that already involved 15 sampled lymph nodes. Prognosis: less than a 10 percent chance of five-year survival.

Dennis

By the age of 29, Dennis had been through chemical dependency treatment six times and failed. When friends or co-workers took him to Alcoholics Anonymous meetings, he would drink before going and then shoot off his mouth at the meeting in the arrogant, critical manner of a drunk. When he returned home, he would drink more. His liver was distended, his job was in jeopardy, his health was failing. Dennis's life was in a shambles. And he wasn't even 30 years old yet.

Kate

Friends and family called Kate and her significant other the perfect couple—young and handsome. Then baby made three. By the time baby was three years old, Kate had learned that bad things can happen behind closed doors. At first, just angry words stung. Then came a slap here, a punch there. Finally, a major altercation sent her to the emergency room. She lied and said one of her gymnastics students had accidentally kicked her. Peering over his glasses with a knowing look, the doctor said, "Only another person's fist could have dislocated this jaw."

Joan

As the thunderstorm approached in the early evening hours, Joan and her 12-year-old daughter Jen were the last ones to leave the campfire. Remembering their Girl Scout training, they gathered up the remaining dry wood and placed it under cover. They held hands as they crossed the top of the granite rock and headed back to their cabin on Minnesota's remote Gunflint Trail. Then a flash of lightning tore through both Joan and Jen, exiting Joan's head in a dramatic 18-foot arc into the sky. They fell to the ground like rag dolls. Despite the heroic efforts of family, friends, and health care professionals, by daybreak, Jen was dead.

THE AFTERMATH

Out of crisis, strength emerges. From agony and despair involving every fibre of spirit and being, it is humanly possible to rebuild courage and vigour.

—ROSEMARY BLACKMON

Crisis came into each of these lives in different ways. For Donna and Joan, it came suddenly, one in the form of an ominous lab report and the other in a flash of lightning. For Dennis and Kate, it came on more insidiously; day after day, year after year, they went through the motions, trying to believe their lives were normal. Dennis continued to drink, and Kate endured the abuse. But for both of them, there was always a nagging urge to find relief. Instead, the next drink beckoned. Or the memories of abuse faded into kissing and making up. Kate and Dennis both delayed their big decision until they were enveloped in so much pain and darkness that they were obliged to give in and reach out for the light.

All four of these people found that light, but they didn't find it on their own. They reached out to others for help—or others reached out to them. And just when they needed it most, they were thankful to find themselves in the company of kindred souls who had been in that same dark valley. The people they encountered in their individual group experiences could honestly say, "I was once as you are, therefore I know what your heart is. I understand."

"There is a tradition in AA that says the only requirement for membership is the desire to quit drinking," says Dennis. "The unwillingness of that group to give up on me, despite all my resistance, was something I had never seen before."

At Joan's first meeting, each group member started out by saying, "We're sorry you're here tonight." Joan was taken aback at first, until she realized the sincerity of their comments—no one would voluntarily choose membership in this group. They understood the pain behind her reason for coming.

Kate's first thought, while still sitting in her car in the parking lot, was that she could just get up and leave if she didn't like the group. Then she watched the other women walking in—young and old, dressed up and in jeans, attractive and well put together, many with young children in tow. She couldn't believe that all these normal-looking women were being abused—just like her.

Donna had barely begun to speak before she started crying at her first group meeting. "But it felt good to have permission to cry, and everybody understood," she remembers. "I needed to share with them every little thing I was feeling, every fear, every pain. I knew that no one would judge those feelings."

When Dennis and Donna and Joan and Kate found their groups, they had turned an important corner. Rather than just treading water or going backward, each one of them had chosen to go forward with life despite the suffering each had endured. None of them did it alone. Instead, each sought out a supportive community of kindred souls and found hope.

Kindred souls don't judge—they understand. Kindred souls don't advise—they listen. Kindred souls don't shame and scold—they forgive. Kindred souls represent a light of hope in the blackest of nights.

> The bird with the broken wing may never soar quite as high again, but often its song is sweeter.
>
> —BRADDUS STREET

Chapter One
What Are Mutual-Help Groups—
And What Can I Expect to Gain?

MUTUAL-HELP GROUPS DEFINED

Historically, people who have shared social, political, medical, or psychological similarities have banded together as a way to meet their needs. Alcoholics Anonymous (AA) is one of the oldest and most successful peer-support networks. For the purposes of this book, the terms *support group, mutual-help group,* and *community* have been used somewhat interchangeably. In general, they all mean the same thing—a group of like-minded individuals who meet together regularly to share and to learn from one another. This definition takes in a broad range of group experiences, including Bible-study groups, which are one of the oldest and most populated forms of mutual-help groups. In many cases, members of a support or mutual-help group share a similar life experience. Often, that life experience—cancer, death of a loved one, chemical abuse, or domestic violence, for example—has created pain and/or difficulty for them. As these groups grow and mature together, they become a community.

LOCATING A GROUP

Finding a mutual-help group that is dedicated to your particular situation may be easier than you think, especially in larger, urban areas. If you have Internet access, let your search engine do the work. Just type in "support groups" and follow the prompts to your area of interest. (For more information on Internet choices, see Chapter Six.) If you aren't hooked up to the Internet, let your fingers do the walking and make some phone calls. Start with your local hospital, community service agency, United Way, YMCA/YWCA, or any social service organization that serves your area. The group you are looking for may be as close as your place of worship.

IS THIS GROUP RIGHT FOR YOU?

Once you have found a group, you could call the group's leader to get more information on exact dates and locations. Also, you could ask the leader the following specific questions to get a sense of how the group operates.

- How many people attend each time, and what is the makeup of the group (age, sex, etc.)?
- How often do they meet? How long are the meetings?
- Where do they meet?
- What is the longevity of the group (that is, is it a time-limited group or an ongoing group)?
- What is the usual format for the meetings?
- What are the leader's qualifications? Is there more than one leader?

The group leader might put you in contact with other group members so you can get a better sense of what to expect. At your first meeting, you will get a sense of the group's atmosphere and will know if it feels right for you. Don't be discouraged if the first group doesn't suit your needs. You usually have other options that may work out better.

WHO LEADS THE GROUP?

Some groups are led by trained facilitators. Others are led by individuals who have personal experience with the group's focus. In general, groups work best when two individuals share the overall leadership. When the group focus is a medical concern, such as cancer, diabetes, or AIDS, group members sometimes prefer to have a health care professional as a cofacilitator so that medical questions can be answered accurately. Grief and bereavement groups are often led by chaplains or bereavement experts. Many groups operate very successfully by sharing the leadership among one another.

SHOULD YOU START YOUR OWN GROUP?

If you are not successful at finding a group, you may need to start your own. The first step might be trying to find a couple of other people who are interested in helping you get the group going. Then you need to look for suitable meeting space in a local church, library, community center, hospital, or social service agency. When you are ready, set a convenient date and time, and publicize your first meeting with public service announcements, press releases, and informational flyers posted in convenient locations. For more information on starting and running a group, please see Chapter Seven, P.S. So You Want to Be a Group Leader.

ESTABLISHING A PURPOSE AND GOALS FOR THE GROUP

> One of the things a community is not is a simple geographical aggregate of people.
>
> —M. SCOTT PECK

When the individuals in a group expend the time and the energy to organize into a community, they usually do so with a list of goals and objectives in mind, which might include:

- To promote understanding and emotional growth through honest group interaction and self-disclosure.
- To encourage group members to focus on their internal resources and to establish realistic expectations.
- To provide a supportive environment that fosters healthy acceptance of each individual's current situation and encourages realistic goal setting for the future.
- To provide an opportunity to share feelings, experiences, and coping strategies with others in a similar situation as a way of assigning meaning to life.
- To see how others deal with similar problems, to gain new information, and to see role models for possible change.

WHAT MAKES GROUPS SUCCESSFUL?

The community created by an ongoing small group provides a place of encouragement and support if these elements are in place: First, the *group is a place to be heard,* so all members must understand how to listen so that each participant feels listened to. Second, the *group represents a place of acceptance*—group members must be nonjudgmental. Third, the *group is a place where one can feel cared for*—the group provides both practical and emotional support. Either way, this caring often represents the spiritual or sacred aspect of the group.

When these three elements are operating successfully, groups of kindred souls end up helping one another in the following ways:

- They encourage one another to honestly express feelings and concerns.
- They listen to and accept one another, without judging.
- They offer each other mutual support when coping with a similar life situation or problem.
- They offer current, accurate information to one another regarding the specific life situation or problem they have in common.
- They help one another find ways to strengthen their problem-solving/coping skills.
- They help one another set goals that result in self-management rather than reliance on others.
- They develop spiritually and emotionally through the ongoing group process.
- They reach out into the larger community in service to others.

What Are the Benefits to Group Members?

I am of the opinion that my life belongs to the community, and as long as I live, it is my privilege to do for it whatever I can. I want to be thoroughly used up when I die, for the harder I work, the more I live.

—George Bernard Shaw

Despite the differences among groups in terms of the reasons they form, the physical, emotional, and spiritual benefits to group members remain remarkably similar. Based on data supplied by members of a variety of supportive communities, the following benefits were reported.

- Acceptance of me as an okay person.
- The feeling that I'm not alone—universality of member experience.
- Knowing I'm not lazy, crazy, or neurotic.
- Validation that what I'm feeling is not "all in my head."
- New friendships and networking possibilities.
- Reinforcement for efforts toward positive action.
- Help with goals.
- Help with feelings of isolation.
- Instillation of hope in what may have seemed a hopeless situation.
- Opportunity to model positive coping behaviors of other members.
- Sense of community and group cohesiveness—we're all in this together.
- Catharsis (release or letting go of emotions).

Research and experience clearly show the psychological benefits of small-group participation. When the group is encouraging, supportive, accepting, expressive, honest, and nonjudgmental, members become comfortable enough to express openly their deepest fears, resentments, and successes. Over time, they grow to trust in the confidentiality and mutual support of the group. When the group has fully evolved into a trusting, safe environment, the healing can begin.

THE FOUR PHASES OF GROUP DEVELOPMENT

Support groups tend to develop most successfully when they cycle through four basic developmental phases. When group meetings are designed to mesh with the natural format of these four phases, group members feel comfortable and benefit from each phase. Even though many support groups are ongoing, they will experience many of the features attributed to the four phases of group development.

Phase 1—In Search of Kindred Souls

During this beginning phase, group members are exploring the group, learning to trust the facilitators, and sensing whether or not it is safe to openly discuss fears and concerns. People are searching for common ground with others who have had similar experiences, or they may be looking for specific information or suggestions on how to deal with their own situation. During this phase, it is important to establish trust, create a comfort level, and provide structure. In Chapter 2, techniques are discussed that relate to each of these three important elements.

Phase 2—In Search of Safety

Somewhere between being strangers and being kindred souls, individuals form a comfortable group relationship and learn how to work together. This transitional phase is further explored in Chapter 3. In this phase, group members are encouraged to carefully evaluate their own needs and to explore ways that peer support can help them get their needs met. A growing sense of closeness helps the group start to uncover the ties that bind them on a more personal level.

During this phase, it is important that facilitators serve as a guide to the group. They can do this by providing equal time for all members and making certain that the group stays balanced. For some people, sharing is not a natural process. The facilitator makes it easier by carefully evaluating each person's needs and personality and finding ways to invite them comfortably into the process. The transitional phase is a time when all members want to know that the group is providing a safe haven. Chapter 3 provides several suggestions to accomplish this purpose, including strict adherence to ground rules such as the confidentiality rule, assurance of the safety of all group members, avoidance of advice giving, and nonjudgmental acceptance of others. Modeling good communication skills is also an important part of this phase.

Phase 3—In Search of Meaning

Once the group members feel comfortable and safe, they are ready to get to the heart of the matter and participate in the real work of support groups. People are now familiar with one another and are involved in sharing sensitive issues and offering caring encouragement to one another. The facilitator now serves as both guide and enabler by raising serious issues and topics, then listening without passing judgment as group members learn to take the risk and honestly share their feelings about these issues.

This phase of exploring for meaning is further discussed in Chapter 4. Individuals assume the roles most comfortable for them. Some people have a tendency to be leaders and others followers. Assertive, outgoing personalities often form a leadership center, or core group, that can be a great asset to a facilitator. The individuals in this leadership center attend most meetings and create a unified, trusting atmosphere that is beneficial for the longevity of the group. Wise facilitators will work with these individuals to good advantage, especially while integrating new members into the group.

No two individuals bring exactly the same needs to the group. During this phase, the group struggles to assign meaning to their experiences, and group discussion will hopefully identify common learnings and coping strategies. These may be tossed out in a random, unorganized fashion. Group leaders then summarize the group's learnings and perhaps identify developing patterns.

Phase 4—In Search of the Future

The last phase in group development often finds people reaching out to the larger community in an altruistic way. For those exiting the group, it is a time of closure. For a group that is staying together, it is a time to reorganize and make new plans. This phase is covered more completely in Chapter 5.

By constantly reinforcing common themes and experiences, group members remember they are not alone, which is one of the of the most important healing qualities of support groups. People find comfort in knowing that other people are thinking the same thoughts and feeling the same feelings.

Through the group's evolution, the facilitator's role shifts from leader to cheerleader. The most effective groups are ones that have become self-governing. Now, the facilitator's main responsibility is helping the group tend to the work at hand. If the group has completed its work together, it's time to find closure and get on with life.

FOUR ROLES OF THE FACILITATOR

Group leaders wear many hats through the four phases of group development. Those hats change with the development of the group. In general, leaders will take on each of the following roles at different stages of the group's development.

The Administrator

The administrator provides and maintains structure for both the meeting and for the group as a whole. The administrator also creatively adapts the format and discussion to suit the unique personality of the group. Once the group has decided on ground rules and group norms, they will look to the facilitator to uphold those rules.

The Nurturer

A facilitator with a genuinely caring and nurturing personality will engender a group that truly helps people. There is no room for phoniness in this position, since a group will pick this up immediately. A nurturing individual creates a warm, hospitable atmosphere where people feel comfortable and accepted. This is done through active listening, acceptance, affection, praise, and understanding.

The Guide

One mission of a successful support group is to take people on a journey of discovery. And the most productive journeys often begin with a clear road map. In addition to being organized and nurturing, a facilitator must be able to guide individuals through this journey and to help them assign meaning to their experience. Many thoughts, feelings, emotions, and life situations will be tossed out for discussion. The guiding facilitator helps individuals sort through what has been discussed to see how it is relevant to their situation.

Because most support groups are ongoing, group members may perceive their situation differently after time. The same scenery can be viewed from a different perspective, depending on a number of variables. For whatever reason, they evolve to a different level. The guide helps direct this journey and point out the differences.

The Enabler

Although "enabler" has developed a negative connotation in recovery circles, an enabler can actually be a very powerful, positive influence in people's lives. The enabler role is one where the facilitator makes it possible for individuals to express their feelings in a protective, safe environment. The enabler raises provocative issues and topics, then listens without passing judgment as group members learn to take the risk and honestly share their feelings about these issues.

❧

In most support groups, the facilitator role evolves as the group evolves. In the beginning, the facilitator is the administrator and carries most of the responsibility for running the group. As the group develops more responsibility for its own direction, the administrative role diminishes. Rather than controlling and directing the group's activity, the facilitator becomes the guide by sensing the group's direction and then assisting movement toward group goals. The facilitator as guide is tuned into the tone of the group, helps members work on their unique concerns, and is responsive to the overall mission of creating a supportive environment for all.

THE HEALING POWER OF A SUPPORTIVE COMMUNITY

Tribal Wisdom—A Historical Perspective

> Coming together is a beginning;
> Keeping together is progress;
> Working together is success.
>
> —JACOB BRAUDE

Working together is, indeed, success. And from that success comes healing.

According to Jim Gordon, M.D., in his book *Manifesto for a New Medicine,* tribal communities have always understood that the way to "make right the things that were wrong" was for people to get together and be honest with each other—in a safe place and in a special way. In their togetherness, they would offer up prayers as a way of invoking the forces of nature and the gods for help. This honest kinship and interaction evolved into a trust level that allowed them to become kindred souls—free to share their most intimate thoughts without fear of reprisal. In essence, they were accepted, with all their flaws and guilts. Kindred souls learn that just saying what needs to be said is a vital part of the healing process. In exposing those innermost fears and thoughts, they quickly learned they were not alone. The tribal behavior described by Gordon is just one example of the beginnings of the self-help movement.

Today, a few tribal societies remain—primarily in undeveloped countries. They still enjoy the comfort of multigenerational extended families who live within shouting distance of one another. They continue to enlist the help of shamans and medicine men and women to bring the tribe together when things are out of balance. But for us today, living in nuclear families, in neighborhoods where we don't even know our neighbors, we have lost all sense of this tribal commune. When our lives are out of balance, we look for new communities of kindred souls to help us heal. And research has now proven the healing power of these new communities.

Research Verifies the Healing

The most profound feelings come from being connected to another human being. People who are involved with others live longer.

—ALLAN LUKS

Back in 1905, Joseph Hershey Pratt, an internist in Boston, was looking for a way to help tuberculosis patients who were too poor to enter sanatoriums. In desperation, he had a brainstorm and decided to bring them together in a small group setting. His hope was that they would find ways to make the illness more manageable by providing support to one another. In so doing, he created one of the first self-help environments, one in which unrelated individuals became kindred souls through their adversity. They understood one another's needs and supported one another during their time of illness, even though they did not have the benefit of institutional support.

In 1989, more than 80 years later, David Spiegel, M.D., a professor of psychiatry at Stanford University School of Medicine, published a landmark study on the effect of psychosocial treatment on patients with metastatic breast cancer. In a very unexpected finding, Spiegel reported that he and his colleagues had studied 86 women who had been randomized into two groups. One group received standard medical treatment only. The other received standard medical treatment plus weekly group-therapy sessions and lessons in self-hypnosis to help control pain. Spiegel found that the women who had been part of a support group lived 18 months longer than the women in the control group.

What was Spiegel's reaction to these findings? "I must say I was quite stunned," he said. Although he had expected to prove that support groups improve *quality* of life, he did not go into the study believing they would also improve *quantity* of life. In fact, he actually initiated the study expecting to refute notions touting the power of mind over disease. Through the whole process, he never created the assumption for his support group that he expected them to live longer due to this intervention. Yet they did—and in addition to longer survival, the women in the support group experienced fewer mood swings and less phobia and pain than their counterparts. What did they do in these groups? They met for 90 minutes per week to express fears, anger, anxiety, and depression, as well as to learn to be assertive with family and physicians. In short, they helped one another in their time of need. "They came to feel that they were experts in living," Spiegel said.

Spiegel's study is backed up by another study using melanoma patients authored by Fawzy I. Fawzy, M.D., out of the University of California at Los Angeles School of Medicine. Like Spiegel, Fawzy initiated the study to assess the value of psychological intervention on the quality of life of individuals with cancer. Early results showed increased vigor and less depression and fatigue among the early-stage melanoma patients.

Six years later, Fawzy discovered another important result of his early psychological intervention. Out of his control group, 10 of the 34 had died, and 3 others had experienced recurrence. But out of his experimental group, only 3 of the original 34 had died and 4 had recurrences. Fawzy's study was not designed to assess survival as an outcome, but the results showed obvious gains for the experimental group. Exactly what was the intervention used? Fawzy's technique was surprisingly similar to the format most support groups follow—90 minutes per week of group meetings that focus on education, stress management, coping skills, and psychological support from staff and other group members.

Although the healing power of small groups has been publicized recently with these studies involving cancer patients, similar findings have occurred in other settings as well. Back in the 1960s, researchers began studying Roseto, a small town in Pennsylvania, that appeared to be inhabited by some of the healthiest individuals in the United States. Despite their typical lifestyle—one that involved smoking, lack of exercise, and stress—this community was thriving. Why? The social structure involved a strong sense of community cohesiveness. People cared about one another with unconditional love and support.

Similarly, Dean Ornish, M.D., a California heart specialist, found remarkable improvements in his heart patients who regularly attended support groups. He concluded that social isolation leads to stress and that the intimacy and connection generated by small groups generates *healing* in the real sense of the word—bringing together and making whole. He concluded that the "ability to be intimate has long been seen as a key to emotional health." This same conclusion was again proven by researchers at St. Luke's-Roosevelt Hospital and Columbia University in New York City: They determined that heart attack patients who lived alone were twice as likely to suffer another heart attack as patients who lived with other people.

In addition to the studies cited, a variety of other independent studies have shown similar results. A synopsis of those studies follows, and the exact listing of the Research Reviews is included as part of the bibliography at the end of the book. All these studies compare self-help participants with nonparticipants, and the material was gathered on multiple occasions over a long period of time.

Mental Health Groups

The Edmunson study reported on a patient-led, professionally supervised social-network-enhancement group for former psychiatric inpatients. After 10 months of participation, when compared with nonparticipants, only one-half as many group participants required rehospitalization. The participants also had shorter average hospital stays.

The Kurtz study showed that 82 percent of 129 members of the Manic Depressive and Depressive Association reported coping better with their illness since joining the self-help group. The longer they were members and the more intensely they were involved with the group, the more their coping had improved.

In the Kennedy study, 31 members of GROW, a self-help organization for people with chronic psychiatric problems, spent significantly fewer days in a psychiatric hospital over a 32-month period than did 31 former psychiatric patients of similar age, race, sex, marital status, and so on. Group members also experienced an enhanced sense of security and self-esteem, decreased anxiety, a broadened sense of spirituality, and increased ability to accept problems without blaming themselves or others.

ADDICTION-RELATED GROUPS

In the Emrick study on Alcoholics Anonymous, the authors conducted a meta-analysis of more than 50 studies. Their conclusions were that AA members stayed sober more if they (1) had an AA sponsor; (2) worked the 12th step of the program; (3) led a meeting; (4) increased their degree of participation over time; and (5) sponsored other AA members. Membership in AA was also found to reduce physical symptoms and to improve psychological adjustment.

The Hughes study compared 25 Alateen members with 25 adolescent nonmembers, all of whom had an alcoholic parent. The study showed that members of Alateen experienced significantly fewer negative moods, significantly more positive moods, and higher self-esteem than the nonmembers.

In a study on the effectiveness of a smoking-cessation program in 43 companies, Jason et al. compared the effects of two smoking-cessation programs in a work setting. One group of 192 workers viewed a television program and used a self-help manual. The other group of 223 workers did the same, but they also attended six self-help group meetings. Initial rates of quitting smoking were significantly higher for the 21 companies that used the self-help groups (41 percent, versus 21 percent in the companies without self-help groups). Three months later, 22 percent of the self-help group continued not to smoke, compared to 12-percent in the companies without self-help groups.

BEREAVEMENT GROUPS

These people—widows and widowers over age 50—whose levels of interpersonal and coping skills were low and who participated in bereavement and self-help groups experienced less depression and grief than did nonparticipants, according to Caserta's study. In a study involving bereaved parents, Videka Sherman showed that parents who attended a Compassionate Friends bereavement self-help group and who were actively involved with group members outside the group increased the parents' comfort in discussing their bereavement and reduced their self-directed anger. Psychotherapy did not have these effects. Compassionate Friends members also reported that the group helped them with their self-confidence, sense of control, and freedom to express feelings.

CAREGIVER GROUPS

Toseland studied two different types of support groups for adult women caring for frail older relatives. One was a peer-led group, and the other was a professional-led support group. Compared to nonparticipants, women in both of the groups experienced significantly greater increases in the size of their support network, increases in their knowledge of community resources, improvement in their interpersonal skills and ability to deal with the problems of caregiving, improvement in their relationships with the care receivers, and decreases in pressing psychological problems.

DIABETES GROUPS

Results of a University of Chicago Medical study of older men with diabetes showed that those who participated in an ongoing, member-led group and who learned self-care techniques were much better off two years later than individuals who didn't take such actions. The men in the group reported being less depressed and less stressed, had more knowledge, and ranked the quality of life higher after two years of group membership. One of the researchers noted that the group leader did not have to be experienced for the session to be valuable.

NEW COMMUNITIES ARE THRIVING

There is a widespread tendency among Americans to get together in small groups—support groups, self-help groups, groups of all kinds. In our fragmented society, where loneliness and isolation are so prevalent, it is encouraging to see so many people reaching out to each other. It's a very hopeful sign for the future.

—GEORGE GALLUP (*NJ MONTHLY,* January 1992)

How are these new communities currently working? Very well, thank you. More than 40 percent of people in America report being members of small groups. An even higher percentage has expressed interest in becoming part of a small group in the future. As these new communities form and grow, the results may seem barely perceptible. But the overall effect could prove to be profound. Every week, often over mediocre coffee and store-bought cookies, these kindred souls show how much they care for one another—by sharing intimate problems, ordinary words of encouragement, recited prayers, details of good and bad weeks, laughter and tears, and genuine acceptance of each person's true identity. And they attend regularly over extended periods of time. Why? In short, because they have found a source of kinship and belonging, as well as a connection to some kind of larger, shared purpose.

In light of these factors, it is no surprise that the self-help movement has grown exponentially. Alcoholics Anonymous, the largest self-help group, now claims over one million members in the United States. People from many different affinity groups have formed support systems, including individuals with addictions, family difficulties, illness or disability, mental illness, bereavement, or alternative lifestyles. Despite the diversity of their individual needs, *developing a community where individuals can help one another* is the center guidepost around which all groups pivot.

> If we make our goal to live a life of compassion and unconditional love, then the world will indeed become a garden where all kinds of flowers can bloom and grow.
>
> —ELISABETH KÜBLER-ROSS

Chapter Two
We Are Not Alone

Through the eyes of our friends
we learn to see ourselves.
Through the love of our friends
we learn to love ourselves.
Through the caring of our friends
we learn what it means to be ourselves completely.

—AUTHOR UNKNOWN

We walked to our cars together, Arne and I. She is a Catholic nun, slight and fair, with a wig of short red hair pulled tightly across her forehead. She speaks in a thick brogue that strongly conveys her heritage. We have completed our second evening of support group together. She has ovarian cancer. I'm the group facilitator.

"I'm not sure of what it is that's happening here," she says, her voice both questioning and excited. "We just talk to one another, say how we feel. It seems simple, really."

"It seems simple," I reply, "but it's magic." I know—because I have been part of groups like this for many years. Magic happens when people learn they are not alone.

She reaches out to me now and touches my arm. "Yes," she answers, quietly and with just a bit of awe. "It is magic. You know that last week, after my first meeting with this group, I slept through the night for the first time since my surgery."

Yes. It is magic. For Sister Arne Malecha, who has always given of herself to care for others, living in the loneliness of her own cancer had become overwhelming. That night, magic happened when this new community of friends cared enough about her to listen to her fears and to respond with encouragement and support.

During her time with this group, Sister Arne's cancer has recurred. When she reported this, the group comforted her and shared their own experiences with recurrence. "When I realized it was back, I felt so helpless. I had done everything I could. And it hadn't worked," she remembers. Yet, thanks to the group, Sister Arne has learned to use the word hopeful *in the same breath as the word* helpless. *"I've seen other people continue to live fulfilling lives despite cancer's recurrence. I can do the same, even though I know I must face this for what it is."*

Sister Arne faces her recurrence one day at a time and continues to fill those days with the activities that provide meaning for her—taking time to visit her mother, reading, and tending to both her earthly and heavenly gardens. Through it all, her newly found circle of kindred souls has given her strength. She knows she is not alone.

EXPLAINING THE MAGIC

There is much satisfaction in work well done; praise is sweet; but there can be no happiness equal to the joy of finding a heart that understands.

—VICTOR ROBINSON

In his book, *A Private Battle,* which chronicled his own experiences with prostate cancer, Cornelius Ryan identified the value of support systems when he said, "I knew her scarcely a week, and yet I knew her very well. Cancer patients have a bond that surpasses a healthy person's understanding."

His observation about cancer patients pertains to all kindred souls who are unified for a common purpose. Most people who join support groups do so because they feel hurt, powerless, or ineffectual, and their loneliness leads them to seek the company of others. When they find the companionship for which they are longing, the bond to which Ryan referred develops quickly and powerfully. Other than the need to develop a connection with others, what causes the magic in a supportive community?

Bonding through Adversity Survivors of major disasters—earthquakes, floods, plane hijackings—often reunite to share their experiences. Holocaust survivors remain in contact with one another through the years. Mutual misfortune creates a bond equal to that of ethnic or familial ties. Although the phrase "misery loves company" has a negative connotation, it should be viewed as a part of the healing process. Being in the company of others who share in your misery can shift a person's attitude from *self-pity* to *self-care.* Just seeing others successfully cope with adversity provides a role model for someone who is trying to understand the process.

Turning Stigma into Courage Society expects perfection. When a person's life situation does not measure up to society's ideal because of illness, divorce, family dysfunction, chemical dependency, abuse, death, or any other variety of socially stigmatizing situations, a person naturally feels alone in that adversity.

People with cancer still suffer social isolation, despite society's attempts to talk more openly about the disease. Individuals with AIDS understand what it feels like to be labeled "the new lepers." Facing such rejection alone is demoralizing. Sharing stories about this stigma—and individual coping strategies for handling rejection—can bolster each person's self-confidence. Being able to laugh at these indignities rather than cry about them results in healing and strength.

Turning the Helpless into Helpers People join a supportive community to help themselves, but they usually end up helping others, as well. Regardless of the reason for joining, a person who once felt helpless usually ends up being a helper to someone else. This is often a surprise silver lining that awaits people who learn to successfully cope with adversity. To aid the healing process, group members assign meaning to their adversity and find ways of turning a negative into a positive. This fuzzy sense of altruism translates into tangible acts of kindness.

Cancer survivors volunteer to help others through programs like Cansurmount and Reach to Recovery. Parents of kidnapped children often create philanthropic foundations to help other parents in the future. When someone is killed by a drunk driver, survivors often dedicate countless hours to organizations like MADD (Mothers Against Drunk Drivers). All these people are turning their helplessness into helping. They are reaching outside themselves and their helplessness to take on a role of helping others.

Back-Fence Wisdom in High-Tech Times Technology may not be a substitute for one-on-one advice from someone who's been there. Just as new mothers tend to trade child-rearing tips over morning coffee, supportive groups offer people a chance to share their own tried-and-true stories with one another. People living with similar adversities may have discovered unique techniques or practical shortcuts for managing a difficult situation. Such folksy bits of advice may not reach the air waves; but practical, face-to-face suggestions from someone who has been through it are delivered in a warmer, easier-to-digest way.

Emotional Release Equals Healing Supportive communities tend to be demonstrative. People touch one another. And because lack of human touch can lead to feelings of isolation and loneliness, these gentle touches, hugs, and pats on the back provide healing and connection. Many people surprise themselves by crying openly at their first group meeting. Seeing others openly showing their emotions in the group environment gives them permission to let down their guard and to admit honestly to their own deep emotional scars caused by their mutual adversity.

As parents, we openly hug and kiss our wounded children. Yet as adults, we often are not as open about our caring and compassion for another wounded adult. The touch of someone who cares is a powerful tool in the healing process. From crying to laughing, hugging to hating, talking to silence, just being in a supportive, understanding environment can bring out pent-up emotions. Many are stunned to discover how much emotion they've been holding in.

When an environment is created in which members feel safe, comfortable, and accepted—and where they can be honest about their feelings—a group's magic can be sustained indefinitely.

OVERCOMING SOCIAL ISOLATION

Perhaps one of life's greatest stresses is the fear that we are alone in the dark.

—RACHEL NAOMI REMEN, M.D., *KITCHEN TABLE WISDOM*

Finding a community of friends—kindred souls—is a way of overcoming our fear of being alone. This gift of friendship is a present you give yourself. When Sister Arne walked into the conference room at St. Joseph's Hospital to attend the support group for the first time, she was giving herself a present—a room full of friends. Even before she started to speak, each person in the room understood the innermost feelings she was about to express. At some time, most had experienced the same thoughts. They had felt isolated in the loneliness of their cancer experience. As they listened to Sister Arne, they accepted her feelings. They supported her concerns. They heard her, without judging her. They nodded their heads in empathy.

That evening, Sister found magic because she had experienced the three basic elements of community: (1) a place where she could be heard, (2) a place where she would be accepted, and (3) a place where others cared for and about her. The magic she felt as a result of this unconditional support stayed with her long after she left the group meeting that evening. And that same magic sustained her through a long night of restful sleep.

When we take the bold step of joining—or forming—a group made up of like-minded individuals, we are giving ourselves a circle of friends. We are developing a kinship that involves sharing honestly of ourselves so that others may grow and learn from us and so that we might grow and learn from them. Each person might enter the room feeling very alone in his or her thoughts and reactions to a life situation. But by taking the risk and joining with others, the loneliness is replaced by togetherness.

LONELINESS MEANS FEELING ABANDONED— JUST WHEN YOU NEED SUPPORT THE MOST

The art of living lies less in eliminating our troubles than in growing with them.

—BERNARD BARUCH

When you are experiencing a crisis or a life transition, it is a time in your life when you need support the most. Yet this is often the time when you get it the least. In most cases, it isn't that others don't *want* to help or be supportive, it's just that they don't understand how you feel—and they don't know what to say or do. They can't empathize with the situation or place themselves in your shoes—*so they say and do nothing.* For you, this may feel like abandonment. As one woman said to Sister Arne: "I just can't imagine how you feel. Sometimes I feel guilty talking to you because all I can think about is how glad I am that it's not me. That's an awful thing to think." It may be an awful thing to think, but it is realistic. When we hear of another person's misfortune, often our first thought is, "I'm so glad that didn't happen to me." We read obituaries with the smug self-assurance and thankfulness that our name is not on the page.

What we fail to realize is that by saying nothing and doing nothing (due to our discomfort), we alienate and socially isolate people we care about. Soon they feel excluded from the everyday flow of normal life. They are on the outside looking in. They withdraw from the world of the healthy and retreat into isolation and loneliness.

"I was at a loss as to where to turn for continued support without being a burden to my friends and my roommate," said Sister Arne that first night. Sometimes it seemed like friends and family would like to go back to things the way they were before . . . before her cancer. But, of course, for Sister Arne, things could never be the same. And the more people acted as if everything was normal again—business as usual—the more lonely and isolated she became. When Sister Arne was with friends and family, she tried to downplay her great concerns. It only deepened her fear and sense of being alone with a frightening secret. The more our real fears are suppressed, the more horrifying they become.

"That first meeting, I remember the friendliness, understanding, and openness of everyone. I felt a noticeable release of tension, and my whole body seemed to relax and soak up the peace and tranquility. I expected more crying, emotional outbursts, and expression of desperate feelings." Although crying and expression of feeling are common in groups, they do not dominate every meeting. Understanding, encouragement, and support are the most common sensations felt at group meetings. People feel cared about in a very special way.

Learning you are not alone also helps dissolve feelings of self-doubt. By talking to others, you realize that your feelings are normal—you're not going crazy—and that others in the group share your feelings—they are also afraid. When you feel isolated, it's probably not because people don't like you. More likely, it's because they truly care about you and are just as frightened as you are.

HOW ARE YOU FEELING?— GETTING PAST SUPERFICIAL COMMUNICATION

I know you believe you understand what you think I said. But I'm not sure you realize that what you heard is what I meant.

—JULIE A. GORMAN

When Sister Arne first spoke up at group, she explained that the reason she came that evening was her loneliness. She did not mean that life itself was lonely. She has a roommate with whom she is very close. And she is part of a cohesive order of nuns, surrounded by people. But she was alone in her cancer experience. When people would ask her how she was feeling, she didn't feel she could honestly respond to them. "Over the weeks and months, I have been responding by saying, 'Oh, I am feeling very good. Just fine.' But some days I'm not feeling very good. I'm not just fine. I needed a place where I could say 'I don't feel so hot today' and know that I am understood."

The group provided just such a place for Sister Arne. During group time, people speak freely about how they are truly feeling. Many have no other place where they can break through the superficiality of everyday conversation. Their family and friends often have heard the same pain repeated far too often. Perhaps they have become nonsupportive and have tired of the topic. This is the point at which Sister Arne found herself that evening. "The more I covered my feelings and stopped talking about them, the more alone I became."

Playing the Glad Game— Pretending All Is Well— Just When You Need Honesty the Most

> Do not free a camel of the burden of his hump; you may be freeing him from being a camel.
>
> —G. K. Chesterton

We tend to feel most alone when others are unwilling or unable to let us share our true feelings. If someone says to us, "Buck up, you're going to be fine, things could be worse," just at a time when we feel like we are drowning in our own grief, the isolation of our grief only intensifies. My mother had a wonderful term for "putting on a happy face"; she called it "playing the glad game." I think it was her way of being accepted—pretending everything was fine in order to make everyone happy and comfortable. But this kind of forced cheerfulness and superficiality is usually not helpful, especially for people faced with a crisis or life transition.

David Spiegel, M.D., in his book, *Living Beyond Limits*, labeled forced cheerfulness "the prison of positive thinking." When we are enduring a life crisis and others are pressuring us to keep our spirits up and to think good thoughts, we feel isolated in this prison of positive thinking. Sister Arne spent a year thinking positive thoughts, primarily because no one would allow her to say anything otherwise. "For over a year, I denied I had cancer by saying 'the cancer'—like it's out there somewhere, rather than belonging to me," she remembers. "Now, I can honestly say 'my cancer' and accept all the fears and negative emotions that accompany the reality of my diagnosis. This has happened since I joined the support group."

Playing the glad game is like pretending that bad things don't happen to good people—that the negative effects of illness and death and abuse and chemical dependency will simply go away if we don't talk about them. Just the opposite is true. Sharing feelings openly in a supportive setting actually helps people to feel more calm and more able to think rationally about what needs to be done for their life situation. Spiegel says that expressing strong feelings in a group setting "has a powerful and positive therapeutic effect."

ACCEPTANCE—JUST AS I AM

Life is not a problem to be solved—but a reality to be experienced.

—KIERKEGAARD

In our everyday lives, we usually do not share honestly and truthfully with most people. Passing in the hallway, at the supermarket, or at a child's baseball game, we simply don't have enough time or concentration to discuss anything deeply important. The weather or the team's batting average are safe discussion topics. When groups form and make a commitment to one another, it presents the members with the opportunity for a deeper level of communication. Within the group environment, members can block out the intrusions of everyday life and can take the time to fully disclose important thoughts and feelings. Implicit in this disclosure is that the group will accept those thoughts and feelings without judging them.

Just knowing you are accepted may be one of the most powerful ways of establishing trust in a group, and often it is what motivates people to remain committed to the group. Every group member expects to be accepted—just as he or she is. Each is seeking encouragement and strength to deal with his or her unique situation. Giving advice or making recommendations is different from being judgmental. People are judgmental when they say: "You are wrong and I am right."

Group leaders serve as role models and create ground rules that set the stage for promoting nonjudgmental acceptance. All group members should draw attention to judgmental statements (in a sensitive way) if they hear them.

THOSE GROUPS ARE TOO DEPRESSING: A COMMON MISCONCEPTION

Only a wounded doctor can heal.

—C. JUNG

A problem kept inside is doubled. A problem shared is divided in half.

—ANONYMOUS

"Don't you find that facilitating a support group is just too depressing?" Group facilitators hear this question often, especially those who work with groups that have come together because of a life crisis like cancer, abuse, or death. The answer to the question is an unequivocal NO. The magic that takes place in a group is the antithesis of depression. Joining together with people who are experiencing a similar pain does not add to that pain. Instead, it dilutes the pain and divides it among the people in attendance, diminishing its power over each individual.

As Carl Jung implied in his quote "Only a wounded doctor can heal," people develop a certain empathetic skill when they have been wounded by illness or crisis. They are sensitive to another person's feelings and know innately how to react. Furthermore, they develop a coping skill through which, by comparison of their situation to that of another, they identify aspects of their struggle that are more positive than those of the next person.

For instance, when Sister Arne's cancer recurred, she was able to take comfort that it was not in a "vital organ," as had been the case with another group member. When she watched young mothers and fathers struggle with the prospect of dying and leaving young children behind, she was grateful that she had chosen a life of celibate service to the church and was not suffering the pain of such a difficult anticipated loss.

CALLED TO ONE ANOTHER: THE ANTITHESIS OF FEELING ALONE

A friend is one
To whom one may pour
Out all the contents
Of one's heart,
Chaff and grain together,
Knowing that the
Gentlest of hands
Will take and sift it,
Keep what is worth keeping
And with a breath of kindness
Blow the rest away.

—ARABIAN PROVERB

When individuals are called to one another, their individual feelings of isolation evaporate. Before joining the group, Sister Arne had felt like there was a glass wall separating her from others. On one side, people seemed to be going about their daily activities without a care in the world. They didn't have cancer. But she did, and she was stuck on the other side of that wall, alone in her fear and isolation.

The group provided safe harbor for Sister Arne's feelings. As a result of being called to one another, each group member responds by providing comfort, bearing one another's burdens, and loving one another through compassion and acceptance. This concept of *one anothering* shattered the glass wall of separation for Sister Arne and let connection—connection with human beings who shared her thoughts and feelings—pour in. "I've learned from others that if I don't speak up about my situation, no one else will. Sharing releases a lot of built-up tension. And humor is good medicine."

Today, she sums up the experience in the following words: "I feel I can share in this group without being a burden to someone. Each time we meet, I feel a noticeable release of tension and sleep so much better that night. I have bonded with each person, and I care about them and want to know more each time we meet. In this group, I have made friends (who will be with me) for the rest of my life."

PHASE 1—IN SEARCH OF KINDRED SOULS

> Friendship is never established as an understood relation. It is an exercise of the purest imagination and the rarest faith.
>
> —HENRY DAVID THOREAU

The experience that Sister Arne described after her first group meeting was a little like falling in love. She had discovered like-minded people who were facing a similar situation and who were filled with hope and possibility. She had finally met people who understood her situation, who accepted her for who she was, and who had expressed genuine caring. In this receptive climate, she could see only the possibilities, not the potential problems.

When you feel like you have *really* been seen and heard, you develop an instant intimacy. But it's good to remember that people bring past disappointments and emotional holes to a group, hoping this new community of kindred souls will help them to forget those disappointments and to fill those holes. Finding your way successfully from this first phase to the fully-developed group requires honesty, commitment, and strong leadership.

GROUPS NEED STRONG LEADERSHIP

During this initial phase, while the group is exploring the possibilities and creating a shared vision, strong leadership is a key ingredient to success. Strong leaders pave the way for committed group members to grow into a lasting community.

Caring—The First Leadership Requirement

Early studies on leadership tried to prove that leaders were born, not made. By testing people on vocabulary, intelligence, and personality, early researchers hoped to show that leadership is inherent and that some people were destined to become leaders. The conclusions? Verbal, organized people with strong personalities tend to be born leaders. *But* anyone who is motivated can *develop* leadership skills.

Whether you aspire to be a group leader or just a group participant, it is good to remember that excellent leadership skills are not the only requirement for building a successful group. The element of caring is equally important. The chief executive officer of a large corporation could be a successful and effective leader without necessarily being a caring individual. This won't work in support group leadership. If you consider yourself to be a caring person, you have satisfied the most important requirement for being a leader.

Valuable Leadership Characteristics

The following list identifies other key qualifications for a successful *group* leader. Keep in mind that the ultimate goal in any group would be to share leadership among the group. If you see yourself reflected in the following list, feel confident that you have the ability to successfully develop and lead a group. Or you can simply keep these characteristics in mind as you interact at your next group meetings.

If you are serious about starting a group, carefully read Chapter Seven of this book, P.S. So You Want to Be a Group Leader. There, you will find specific tips for helping your group to succeed from the very first meeting.

A good leader is . . .

A people person with strong verbal skills Good facilitators genuinely enjoy being with people. Because of this, they are able to engage all members of the group and create an environment that leads to strong group interaction.

Experienced in group dynamics or leadership For an inexperienced facilitator, this book provides the basic building blocks for developing successful groups. A new facilitator might feel more comfortable in the initial stages of a group's development if he or she could connect with someone experienced in group dynamics and facilitation who would serve as a cofacilitator.

Organized A successful group follows a certain format each time, which requires planning and organizing. A successful facilitator comes prepared, adheres to a certain structure, and provides strong leadership, particularly in the group's formative stage.

A good listener Listening skills are covered in more detail later in the book because they are an integral part of a group's success. Skilled leadership means setting aside personal biases and prejudices in order to listen to each group member individually with fresh, nonjudgmental ears. To do this, a facilitator must be able to accept individuals with differing abilities and personalities.

Able to ask questions, to summarize, and to keep a discussion building in the needed direction The leader is the conduit for the group's discussion, a role quite different from that of a teacher or a lecturer. A teacher has a set lesson plan with a goal of disseminating certain information. Leaders rely on the group to provide the lesson plan. This means listening carefully to what each individual says, then summarizing the information and asking the right questions to keep the discussion building in a certain direction.

Capable of resolving conflict Hidden conflict can inhibit group development. On the other hand, conflict can be helpful and constructive if it is brought out into the open. Skilled leadership means being able to cope with open conflict when it arises as well as to elicit hidden conflict when the group is avoiding it. Groups that encourage complete honesty and welcome healthy conflict should move smoothly through the phases of development.

Gifted with a sense of humor Leaders who can inject humor in a sensitive and caring fashion are a real asset to any group. Humor in a group setting is contagious, even when dealing with very difficult or serious issues. Humor can be healing. When people feel the camaraderie of others facing a similar situation, they find it easier to laugh at themselves. People who see the light side of things usually cope better.

Committed to the value of peer support If facilitators believe in the healing power of peer support, they will naturally show excitement and their commitment to the group's success. A facilitator's enthusiasm will be one of the great motivators for other group members.

GROUPS NEED STRUCTURE

In Phase 1, structure and strong leadership are necessities for building cohesiveness and for helping group members to feel safe. A common misconception about small groups is that the individual group members are responsible for what happens and that structured leadership is not so important. Just the opposite is true, especially in the beginning. A truly successful group begins with a strong leader. That person structures the environment and gently leads the group toward the eventual goal of self-leadership.

When structure is missing, the group could be likened to a rudderless ship—lacking direction, it may spin in circles indefinitely, getting nowhere. Conversely, a strong leader is the rudder that guides the group and provides direction. Members learn to feel safe when they can rely on one or two leaders to provide guidance based on the unique needs of the group.

Starting Off on the Right Foot

When you walk into the meeting room that first time, you are entering with certain expectations. If the group fulfills those expectations, you will probably go back. Almost universally, people want to feel *noticed, comfortable,* and *accepted.* Whether you are an existing group member or a leader, if you make an effort to satisfy those three wants of new members, you will have a high probabilty of success.

In a group's formative stages, members are exploring the group, learning to trust the facilitators, and sensing whether or not it is safe to openly discuss fears and concerns. They are looking to establish a common ground with others who have had similar experiences. They may be seeking specific information or suggestions on how to deal with a specific problem. At this time, three important elements are *structure, trust,* and *finding a comfort level.*

Establishing Group Structure

One important objective in Phase 1 is to establish a structure from the very beginning. In general, every time a group gets together, it might want to adhere to the following general outline:

Start and End on Time. Leaders can develop a safe, protective environment for new group members by adhering to a certain set of group norms, beginning with a predictable start time and end time for every group meeting. If the advertised start time is 7:00 P.M., then the meeting should start right at 7:00, even at the risk of having people arrive after the meeting has started. This establishes a clear expectation for everyone. Activities should be planned carefully so the meeting can also close at the announced time.

Follow Ground Rules That Suit the Group's Needs. Ground rules are important for two reasons. First, they set a disciplined tone and give the message that the group is serious in its intentions. Second, they help set group norms by clearly stating what is and what is not acceptable. If people disobey the ground rules, they can be reminded of the rule in a nonthreatening way.

> *In one of my groups, we had a woman who truly was unable to participate effectively in a group. By this, I mean she attended the group primarily to tell her story (on a continuing basis), to relate how and why she had been wronged, and she essentially used the group as a place to "vent her spleen." Because we are an open group*

and do not restrict attendance (although many in the group regarded her behavior as bothersome), the behavior had to be tolerated.

A ground rule stating "Each member may speak for 10 minutes—no more—unless they are in crisis" saved us many times. Even though it was uncomfortable to remind this woman of the 10-minute rule, it was a group norm that had been agreed on by all members—including her!

Generally, a group respects and "owns" ground rules if participants have the opportunity to suggest rules and to decide which ones will be used. Many groups adopt some or all of the following ground rules.

- Group always begins and ends on time.
- Confidentiality and respect for each other's privacy.
- No side conversations between group members are allowed during the meeting.
- All feelings are acceptable, whether positive or negative.
- No one monopolizes the conversation—the "10-minute rule."
- One person speaks at a time.
- Each group member is accepted without judgment.
- Sharing with others is encouraged, not required.
- Listen carefully. Give advice sparingly.

Introduce Group Facilitator(s) Facilitators begin by introducing themselves and by stating their personal connection to the group's purpose and their reason for becoming a facilitator. Personalizing this introduction helps create a comfort zone for members. Good eye contact makes people feel welcome and noticed.

Go Over Housekeeping Details At the first meeting and at subsequent meetings when new people have joined, the group should cover general housekeeping items, which may include the following:

- Details regarding parking and handicap access information.
- Location(s) of rest room(s).
- Dates and times of upcoming meetings and any dates you will NOT meet.

Cooperatively Develop Opening and Closing Rituals Groups with a religious component can close each meeting quite naturally with a prayer. However, even groups that are nondenominational also benefit from opening and/or closing rituals. Many groups use a centering exercise such as deep breathing, meditation, light imagery, or affirmations. Such exercises serve to awaken intuition, to clear the emotions, and to relax the body.

Last October, Donna H. and I started a new group for women with recurrent cancer. We call it Affirming Life. At our first meeting, we opened with a very brief breathing and relaxation exercise. Deep breathing and relaxation are one way to make the transition from most people's typical hectic pace to what you hope will be a more thoughtful, peaceful environment for the one or two hours you are together.

At the end of our meetings, we allow five to ten minutes to read a short story to the group. For our first meeting, I used Rachel Naomi Remen's "Gift of Healing" from her book Kitchen Table Wisdom, *a perfect message for that first meeting. Establishing a ritual beginning and ending provides structure and helps the group feel safe. After several months of meetings, I have read almost all of Remen's book out loud. The group looks forward to those stories with anticipation.*

Groups Need Honest Communication

> One of the definitions of community is an aggregate
> of people who have made a commitment to learn
> how to communicate with each other at an ever
> more deep and authentic level.
>
> —M. Scott Peck

Honest communication is vital to small groups. Communication includes relationship building, self-expression, listening, being listened to, receiving, feeling, and speaking. For honest communication to develop, group members must speak honestly and directly with one another, speaking their own truth rather than attempting to interpret someone else's. Honest communication allows a group to deepen their intimacy and is the primary way a group grows to full maturity. Five ways group members can develop honest communication are: (1) using "I" statements, (2) listening without judging, (3) speaking directly to the other person, (4) learning to honor moments of silence, and (5) paying attention to nonverbal communication signals.

Use "I" Statements

> Look well into thyself; there is a source of strength
> which will always spring up if thou wilt always look
> there.
>
> —Marcus Aurelius

When we use "I" statements, we own and take responsibility for our own thoughts, feelings, and actions. Group members can't read one another's minds. By consciously using "I" statements, group members can guard against being misunderstood or having their words misinterpreted. By using "I" instead of "you" to begin a sentence, the speaker takes responsibility for his or her feelings rather than placing the burden on someone else; for example, "I felt hurt when you said such and such," rather than "You really hurt me." Although the two sentences are similar, the implications are quite different.

Listen without Judging or Giving Advice

It is possible that in the realm of human destiny, the depth of man's questioning is more important than his answers.

—ANDRE MALRAUX

One of the most tempting responses during a group meeting is that of offering advice or providing answers. This fact holds true for both facilitators and group members. We're all anxious to give our own personal brand of advice to someone faced with a difficult dilemma. Although there are times when such advice is helpful—and the person might actually benefit from your suggestion—in most cases, people don't come to a group looking for advice. In fact, just the act of sharing often helps people to see the situation more clearly and leads them to their own personal solution—without outside help.

Communication happens when group members concentrate on closing their mouths and opening their ears. Active listening shows people that you care, especially when you carefully listen for both *content and feeling*. When people are sharing feelings and they sense that you are listening rather than judging, they feel accepted, respected, and understood. Remember, all feelings are acceptable.

Speak Directly

> One of the most terrible responsibilities of the world
> is that of really being present, of being a presence
> for the other. We cannot achieve dialogue by an act
> of will, for dialogue is a genuinely two-sided affair.
>
> —MAURICE FRIEDMAN

In a group meeting, look directly at and speak directly to the other person. Instead of saying, "Pat brought up a good point and I wanted to add something," look directly at Pat and say, "I thought your point was very interesting because it reminded me of a time in my life when . . ."

Similarly, if you have an issue with another group member, don't take the easy way out by going behind that person's back and discussing the issue with someone else. Take the grievance to them personally and work it out between the two of you.

Appreciate the Power of Silence

> Silence, then, could be said to be the ultimate province of trust; it is the place where we trust ourselves to be alone; where we trust others to understand the things we do not say; where we trust a higher harmony to assert itself.
>
> —PICO IYER

Just as words communicate a strong message, silence can be equally as powerful. Consider how you feel when someone gives you "the silent treatment" as a form of punishment. In the same way, silence can be a powerful positive message. Quakers call it an "opening to spirit." Native Americans use silence at the end of a meeting to help them resolve conflict.

Silence provides time for personal reflection and helps people to absorb and integrate what has been said. It also gives group members time to observe what has been happening and perhaps switch directions, if necessary. Silence is intimate—it allows members to get centered and to hear their inner voice. Be still and let silence do its work!

Even though I had been facilitating groups for years, the first few meetings of any new group are always question marks. How many people will show up? Will they all want to share? What will we do with the silent moments? After our first Affirming Life group meeting, I shared my concerns about these long silences with Donna. She reminded me that sometimes the hardest part is to sit in silence and not fill the void with forced words. From that silence will emerge new insights.

The next week, I listened to Donna's advice. When the silence arrived, I fought back my first impulse—to provide a link from one topic to the next. I simply sat in silence. The next person to speak was Pat, and she revealed a very moving description of how and why she suspected her recurrence. She had never told anyone this story before. Donna was so right. Closing my mouth—opening my ears and listening to the silence—revealed new insights for all of us.

Pay Attention to Nonverbal Communication

In general, human communication usually breaks down into the following components: 7 percent verbal, 20 percent tone of voice, 23 percent facial expression, and 50 percent body position. Just think, only 7 percent is actually verbal. That proves that it's not what you say, it's how you say it! These percentages point out that dishonest communication may be easier to spot than you think. If you are saying one thing, but your tone of voice, facial expression, and body position are saying something else, the group will pick up on the dissonance.

Communication is most effective when group members are aware of all four components: eye contact, facial expression, tone of voice, and body position. Everyone should distinguish between *what* is being said and *how* it is being said, which can be colored by tone of voice or verbal expression and perhaps evoke a totally different response. If a member's verbal and nonverbal messages don't match, he or she is not engaging in authentic communication.

NONVERBAL COMMUNICATION SKILLS

The following communication techniques are some of the most successful ways to get a message across without using words.

Eye Contact The eyes often send the first important nonverbal message between people. Avoiding eye contact or shifting eyes signals avoidance. On the other hand, constant eye contact can be unsettling and overly aggressive and can make some people uncomfortable. When people are discussing uncomfortable topics, they may reduce the anxiety of that discussion by frequently breaking eye contact, closing their eyes, or blinking. When people are making good eye contact, they signal that they are paying attention to the speaker. People want to be understood, and they can feel that the listener cares about what they are saying when eye contact is maintained.

Facial Expression Facial expression reflects emotion. Just by studying a person's face, you can often tell if they are happy or sad, nervous or relaxed, anxious or self-satisfied, hostile or cheerful. You might check with that person to verify if their facial expression is indicative of their mood—"Bill, your brow is furrowed, which says to me that you're worried about something. Am I right?" This gives the person a chance to immediately respond. If you are right, you can pursue this line of thought. Group members can also *give* information through facial expression and should be consciously aware of their own mannerisms as they look at and talk to one another. Are you smiling or serious? Are you tense or relaxed? Your face shows your emotions.

Voice Inflection A voice's tone, volume, and pitch help us identify the hidden nonverbal messages in what someone is saying. In general, a loud voice might imply anger or hostility, whereas a weak voice can sound passive and compliant. Someone speaking in a monotone implies boredom or depression. In a similar way, a person can use voice inflection to indicate how strongly he or she feels about something.

Body Position A listener's physical position tells the speaker just how involved and interested he or she really is. Leaning forward in a chair shows interest and encourages the speaker to keep talking. Posture should be open and relaxed, yet alert, with arms, hands, and head comfortable, not rigid. If possible, the listener should face the speaker squarely rather than with the head turned to the side. As people talk, depending on the emotion and the content being expressed, the listener can encourage with gestures such as nodding the head or reaching out a hand to indicate positive feelings.

GROUP CHALLENGES AND CONFLICTS

Should you shield the canyons from the windstorms, you would never see the beauty of their carvings.

—ELISABETH KÜBLER-ROSS

The challenges and conflicts of a group are proof that it is a diverse community of individuals learning to understand one another and collectively grow. One sign of a healthy, ongoing group is the ability of the members to successfully manage the inevitable challenging personalities and group behaviors that are bound to emerge. Gaining some measure of control over those challenges is prudent, or these people may end up controlling the direction in which the group is headed.

The first, catch-all solution starts in the group planning stages when you decide on how to structure the leadership. Groups that are facilitated by two individuals handle challenges and conflicts more easily. You can often "divide and conquer" when difficult situations arise.

The next section describes specific challenging behaviors (both personal and group) with possible ways of handling them. When all group members work together with the leader to correct some of these challenges as they occur, many potential sources of irritation can be eliminated. But groups are unpredictable. Some groups could encounter *all* of these behaviors at the first meeting. On the other hand, a leader may be fortunate and never need to refer to this section of the book at all. If so, congratulations are in order!

Challenging Personalities

Every group will have its mix of personalities—soft-spoken and gregarious, passive and aggressive, happy and angry, depressed and overly optimistic—and some people who are just plain normal. This distinct mix of personalities will eventually translate into a unique group dynamic. For instance, if your group is comprised of many outgoing, opinionated individuals, you may need to watch for monopolizers or advice givers and to develop ground rules that make certain that all group members are given equal time. On the other hand, a group of introverted, somewhat insecure individuals may require some coaxing to get them to openly interact.

Whatever the mix of your group, you might expect to see one or more of the following people show up at your door.

THE QUIET MEMBER

People who are shy or quiet by natural disposition are not destructive to the group, but they may need some encouragement to participate in group discussion. Everyone is different, and some need more time or help in self-disclosure. Silence is not good or bad, but it can be misunderstood by other group members. The following ideas may help:

1. Especially in the early group-formation phase, silence is perfectly acceptable, and your ground rules probably state that it is okay to pass. Group members should encourage the quiet member, not manipulate. Make certain everyone feels welcome.

2. At the first meeting, you might divide your group into pairs for the icebreaker (Discussion Guide #1 at the end of this section on challenges and conflicts). A smaller grouping makes discussion easier for some people.

3. Attempt to draw out each person's personal interests. Go around the group asking questions, but give the quiet person time to think before responding. Then listen attentively to what he or she has to say.

4. Try to spend time with quiet people before or after the meeting, reassuring them that they are not the only ones who are uncomfortable speaking up.

5. Find a time where it seems natural for the quiet person to share something, then ask a question. Sometimes a direct question helps a person feel affirmed and noticed. When he or she answers, respond positively.

6. Try to get the rest of the group involved in drawing the person out as well. Watch closely for nonverbal cues indicating that the person is interested in the conversation, for instance, a nodding of the head or a note of interest in the eyes.

The Monopolizer

Some participants talk more than others. Occasionally, these talkers tend to monopolize the conversation so that others are unable to talk. When this happens, it doesn't take long for people to become discouraged or silently irritated about their group experience.

It seems that almost every group has at least one monopolizer, which makes it even more important that group members are watchful and understand how destructive this behavior can become. Monopolizers, if left to their own devices, can destroy group cohesiveness very quickly. The following ideas may help.

1. At the very first group meeting, your Ground Rules can discourage anyone from dominating the group. Each group member should be held accountable for his or her own behavior and should be sensitive to the danger of monopolizing.
2. Include the "10-minute rule" in your ground rules (see page 46). Any members who break this rule can be gently reminded about it.
3. Monopolizers are encouraged by eye contact. For this reason, you may wish to limit your eye contact with people who have a tendency to dominate group time.
4. Don't respond to the monopolizers' comments if they continue to carry on too long. A response will encourage them to continue.
5. Don't be afraid to break in, particularly to praise one of the monopolizer's statements. Then raise a new question and ask for a response from other members of the group.

The Joker

This person (often a man) is the life of the party and can make a joke out of anything just to get a laugh. He or she genuinely enjoys a good joke and loves to be in the spotlight. The joker might also feel a certain tension within the group setting and find that joking is the only way to relieve it. In many ways, this person can provide comic relief, with the humor being somewhat of an icebreaker for other nervous individuals in the group. The following ideas may help deal with the joker:

1. The joker can be encouraged, if desired, by complimenting the person's wit.
2. When time is limited and the comments are inappropriate, group members might ignore the joker's comments and continue the discussion.
3. If the joker persists, and any group member considers the behavior to be inappropriate, you might make a statement such as: "There's a time for work and a time for play, and right now we need to work."

THE ANGRY MEMBER

Expression of emotions is encouraged in small groups. Because support groups often are organized around crisis or loss, group members have good reason to feel angry. They have lost control of part of their life and their environment. In addition, they may be frustrated by how hard they have tried, with little or no success, to find comfort. This group environment may be one of the only places where individuals feel safe venting their anger.

As long as anger is balanced against other positive group experiences and doesn't dominate the group, people should be sensitive to angry feelings and allow individuals to vent. But once that anger has been released, most people are able to move on. If someone's anger doesn't dissipate with time or if the anger becomes dangerous or hostile and is directed inappropriately, you should feel justified intervening and redirecting that person's behavior. The following suggestions may help.

1. Before you react, try to examine the reasons for the person's anger—was it something that was said within the group? If so, put yourself in the angry person's shoes and try to see that point of view.
2. Under no circumstances should you allow the anger to be directed at someone in the group.
3. If individuals exhibit a constant pattern of anger with no counterbalancing positive responses, a referral may be in order.

THE IMPOSING/DOMINATING MEMBER

This person's suggestions and opinions are *always* right, and he or she will be the first one to speak up and tell you—my way or the highway! This behavior quickly intimidates a group. Others become reticent to speak for fear of being judged by the "expert." The dominator has a hard time with silence and will step in and lead whenever possible. Some ideas for handling the dominator include:

1. Develop ground rules that speak to the issue. For instance, two ground rules that would apply are: (1) We listen with understanding but don't judge or offer solutions. (2) There are no right or wrong answers, only discussion.
2. Remind everyone in the group to be watchful of his or her own behavior when it comes to fixing or judging someone else. We are all guilty.

THE FIXER

Many people believe that the way to help another person is to fix his or her problem. Once group members get to know one another and learn about each individual's situation, the ideas start flowing. Everyone has his or her own personal fix for the other person's problem: Change doctors. Kick the bum out of the house. Just say no. Apologize and make peace. Start going to more AA meetings . . . The potential solutions are endless. Unfortunately, a solution usually isn't the response most people are looking for. The following guidelines may help group members work around this situation.

1. Remember that you are are together to support and to encourage, not to advise or to fix.
2. Express appreciation when people offer suggestions, but stress that any attempt to rescue someone is not productive.

Challenging Group Dynamics

Sometimes simple group dynamics can be challenging. You can either create a learning experience out of the incident or simply try to ignore it and and try to get your group back to order. The following group problems are a few of the most common, but others may arise as well. There are no right or wrong solutions to these problems. You know the group best, but you may find guidance in the suggestions that follow.

CHATTING WITH YOUR NEIGHBOR

Side conversations can be very disruptive to group dynamics. Other group members feel excluded and offended. These conversations appear personal and secretive rather than all-inclusive and shared. The following ideas may help.

1. Some people are unaware of how disruptive this activity is, or they have never been a member of a group where it was not tolerated. You may prevent these conversations by establishing a ground rule from the very beginning that prohibits chatting with your neighbor.
2. If people forget the ground rule or can't control their impulse to talk, the leader should intervene immediately, interrupt the conversation, and ask the individuals if they would share their discussion with the entire group.

THE SILENT GROUP

Any group has the potential to become tired and apathetic. This lethargy can create frustration when you are anxious for the group members to bond. Sometimes when the group is silent, they may have reached a plateau in their level of intimacy. They may be looking for direction on how to take their group relationship a step further.

At this point, strong leadership may once again be a key factor. When the leader must reassume the role of administrator/director of the group, personal disclosure often is the best way to get a group talking at a deeper level. If the leader tells a personal story that involves self-disclosure and if the story relates to the subject at hand, it may pull the group back in and create conversation.

This is a time to display enthusiasm and energy and perhaps to pose questions to the group that invite response. The leader could also throw the problem back out to the group by posing a question such as: "It doesn't feel like we're getting much accomplished tonight. I wonder if any of you can think of a reason why and share it with the rest of the group."

Discussion Guide #1
Getting to Know One Another
Who Are We?

GROUP EXERCISE

The purpose of this exercise is to provide a more in-depth introduction of group members to one another. Group members pair up (preferably not with the person they came with) and interview one another using the interview form provided at the end of this section. At the end of the interview period, each person introduces his or her partner to the group. If the group has an odd number of members, the group leader participates in the exercise to give everyone a partner.

DISCUSSION

Once the individuals have introduced one another, group leaders might pose the following questions and put the answers on an overhead, a flip chart, or a chalkboard.

- How did you learn about this group? What is your reason for coming?
- How many are experiencing a life change or a crisis personally? How many are here to support that person, either as a friend, partner, or caretaker?
- What do you hope this group will do for you?
- What do you consider your greatest challenge?

SUMMARY

Once the group has answered these questions, the leaders summarize the responses on one overhead or on the chalkboard. Ask group members for permission to prepare a summary of their responses that could be used as a handout at the next session. Preparing this list of responses is a good way to personalize this group as being unique, with its own set of challenges and hopes.

After this meeting, facilitators and group members should have a general idea of:

- Why group members are attending.
- What percentage are personally experiencing crisis versus people who are there to support others.
- A list of hopes.
- A list of challenges.

Discussion Guide #2
Discovering the Power of Words

Words have the capacity to harm and the capacity to heal. Some words used to describe people who are sick, chemically dependent, or simply different have become commonplace in our vocabulary. That doesn't make them right. In fact, using these words repeatedly may have a significant negative impact on how these individuals view themselves. Conversely, by consistently using more positive descriptive words, individuals may begin to actually feel more positive about who they are and what has happened to them.

GROUP EXERCISE

Open the exercise by asking group members one or more of the following questions, and encouraging everyone to participate:

- As a part of living through this life change or crisis, what words have you used to describe yourself? Have those words changed over time?
- How have you heard others describe people in your situation? in the media? in general conversation?
- Do you think that the words people use have an effect on how you view yourself?

Leader's Responsibility: As a group leader, you may want to prepare for discussing this concept by clipping articles from newspapers, magazines, or journals or by recounting television or radio news stories that depict people as "victims" or "sufferers." You could also come prepared with a personal remembrance of how someone in your acquaintance fell victim to the negative power of words. The more examples you can provide of the concept, the easier it will be for the group members to understand and to enter into the discussion.

DISCUSSION

Words often point us in the direction we go, so we should choose our words carefully. If we constantly talk about being sick, we invest our illness with a lot of power, and we may stay sick. But if we begin to say things like "I'm getting better," we add positive energy to our words and point our actions in the right direction. The act of defining is an act of power. We should encourage one another to define ourselves rather than relying on others (health care professionals, media, family, etc.) to describe us and what we need.

Words are tools. They work at building our future, whether we are conscious of it or not. Hand out the following list of words and begin a discussion that compares the impact of each harming word and each healing word on individuals within the group. Conclude with the importance of putting *people* before *affliction*.

Words That Heal	Words That Harm

Experiencing ⎯⎯⎯⎯
  (a life crisis)
	Suffering ⎯⎯⎯⎯
	  (a life crisis)

Brain injury	Brain damage
Survivor	Victim

Words That Heal	Words That Harm
Client	Patient
Recovering alcoholic	Drunk
Abused	Loser chooser
Physically challenged	Cripple
Acceptance	Put up with
I care	Get over it
I'm sorry	Don't worry—everything will be okay

(Add words of your own!)

SUMMARY

In general, words that are perceived as *helpful* usually are empowering and positive, show genuine compassion, assure continuing support, and convey hope. Words that are perceived as *harmful* usually suggest lack of control, are trite or sound like platitudes, disregard feelings, are cold and cynical, or destroy hope.

After this meeting, group members should have an idea of:

- The powerful impact of words, both positive and negative.
- The value of speaking positively about yourself and others.
- Words to use and words to avoid when talking to other survivors.
- The importance of being a *survivor, not a victim.*

INTERVIEW FORM

Getting to Know You Exercise
Discussion Topic #1

1. What is your partner's name?

2. Is your partner experiencing a life crisis or here to support someone experiencing a crisis? What is their relationship?

3. How did your partner learn about our group?

4. What hobbies does your partner enjoy?

5. What does your partner hope to gain by becoming part of our group?

6. What is your partner's greatest challenge today?

EVALUATION

This evaluation form may be used at the close of any meeting.

1. Did you like the topic chosen for discussion?

   Yes ___   No ___

   Comments:

2. Did you learn anything new from the discussion?

   Yes ___   No ___

   Comments:

3. How do you intend to use what you learned here in your daily living?

   Comments:

Chapter Three
People Needing People

To be present to one another, to be a true friend, means to be forever on call, forever open, forever willing to be involved in the friend's troubles.

—Douglas V. Steere

Jackie, a fine-featured, small-boned, and handsome woman just past 50, joined our support group soon after her husband Richard was diagnosed with a rare, terminal, primary bile duct cancer. High school sweethearts, they were married and started a family when Jackie was 20. At the time of diagnosis, their two children, David and Terry, had completed college and were both living out of state. For the past 25 years of their marriage, Jackie and Richard have lived in a large brick home on a remote, heavily wooded property in Afton. The house is situated beside a meandering creek, and the water's soothing sounds murmur peacefully through every open window in the house. Yet it was only in Richard's last few months of life that he sat still long enough to watch and hear the beauty of his surroundings.

Sheri is a tall woman, just past 30, with a bright smile and even brighter blue eyes. As she tells it, she and her husband Randy were the perfect couple with the perfect marriage. After meeting on a blind date, it was love at first sight. Seven months later, they were engaged—eleven months later, married. Zachary, baby number one, arrived the next December. Then came building the new house and getting ready for Adam, baby number two, in October of 1994. Two weeks after Adam's birth, Randy was diagnosed with a rare cancer in his spinal cord. They were convinced that surgery would be the cure. But when the cancer recurred a year later, Sheri told Randy she needed help. She wanted to join a support group. He balked at first, but then agreed to go for her sake.

Jackie struggled, and the group struggled with her, as she watched Richard fight—and finally fade. During this time, Randy had two more surgeries and many rounds of chemotherapy. For awhile the tumors receded, only to return again and again. Through it all, Sheri and Randy supported and comforted Jackie in her 11-month struggle toward Richard's death. And during that time, Sheri began to see a bit of herself in that struggle. How long will it take? When will we know the end is near? How can we learn to face this and talk about it? The similarity of their experience was forging a bond between these women, even though they had barely begun to recognize it.

After Richard died, Jackie continued to attend the group. Just as they had supported her in her struggle with Richard's cancer, they now supported her in her grief and her adjustment to life alone. She announced that her number one goal was to just stay busy.

At Christmas time, the group exchanged names and addresses for sending notes and cards. Only then did Jackie and Sheri realize that they lived only two miles from one another. That meant they could drive to group together. When more surgery made it difficult for Randy to drive sometimes—or if he simply didn't feel up to attending—the two women came together. In between *time, Jackie often watched the two boys when Sheri needed a break.*

Then the unexpected happened. Sheri announced she was expecting their third child—a risky and unanticipated occurrence given that Randy was still on chemotherapy. The group again encouraged the couple with the excitement and anticipation that should rightfully surround the birth of a new baby. During Sheri's 36th week of pregnancy, Randy had more spinal surgery, which put him in a wheelchair. Now he couldn't drive, and they began worrying about getting to the hospital and about labor and delivery. Jackie immediately volunteered to be both driver and labor coach. For her, it made perfect sense—she lived close by, she had time on her hands, and she wanted to help.

Early the morning of June 24, Jackie drove Sheri and Randy to the hospital. She sat with Sheri, rubbed her back, and helped her breathe. Finally, at 3:34 P.M., Randy and Jackie witnessed the birth of Miranda Nicole—the miracle of Randy. In a matter of two years, these strangers had become relatives. And Miranda Nicole has a third grandmother, Grandma Jackie.

BALANCING SELF AND OTHERS

The very fundamental of happiness is that its possession comes from the fullest realization of self in terms of achievement—and most often in behalf of others.

—HUGHSTON M. McBAIN

Jackie came to support group the first time because she needed help. She had been Richard's primary source of emotional support all through their marriage, and she knew he would expect her to do the same during his illness. That necessitated a way of finding support for herself. Richard was a private man who would never attend the group himself, but he understood that the group experience was helping Jackie and giving her emotional strength to deal with the gravity of their situation.

"I was looking for so many answers when I first joined," Jackie remembers. "I needed to know about treatment, side effects, and alternative therapies. I searched for answers to communication problems I was having with his family and our friends. I needed spiritual support as we faced the prospect of death. I felt very needy at that time, and the group was always willing to share their thoughts and experiences."

As time went on, the group gave Jackie strength and helped her learn how to mobilize her resources and face the situation with courage. The more her needs were met, the more she could help Richard. And the more the group helped her, the more Jackie wanted to give back. Developing a closer relationship with Sheri and Randy was an outgrowth of all that Jackie had gained through group support.

"Once you have been through this experience, once you have watched a loved one die, there seems to be a need to share what you have learned and help others who are going through the same thing. We received so much love and support from family and friends. I, personally, received incredible strength and encouragement from my group. I wanted to repay people in any way I could."

For Sheri, Jackie was a gift from heaven. She was a sounding board when it seemed impossible for Sheri to get through another day faced with the physical and emotional challenge of juggling caretaking chores among the children and Randy. Jackie could confirm for Sheri that her feelings were normal—that she wasn't going crazy. She comforted Sheri when Randy seemed overly demanding and resentful, reminding her that Richard had lashed out at her in a similar manner—we always hurt the ones we love. Sheri was living each day in the abyss of the unknown. Because Jackie had already walked a similar journey, had lived through that unknown and survived, she knew many of the road markers. Although Sheri's situation was bound to be different, the emotions were the same.

"Jackie can anticipate how I am feeling," says Sheri. "She calls and offers to watch the kids just at the time when I need her most."

Because she remembers how hard it was for her to ask for help, Jackie takes the initiative to call Sheri. "When you're at the lowest point—at the time when you need help and support the most—you are too tired or depressed to reach out," remembers Jackie. "I'm at a place where I have time on my hands. To watch Sheri's kids and give her some peace is the least I can do."

Jackie and Sheri's situation shows how group development evolves from getting to know one another into a deeper connection where you discover how much people need people.

DISTINGUISHING THINKING FROM FEELING REVEALING TRUE EMOTIONS

The most relevant source of information for most people is their own experience and their reflection upon that experience.

—SIDNEY HOOK

Thinking and feeling are quite different human reactions to events. When you are faced with a life crisis, your *thinking* brain engages in a cerebral process of gaining information, forming opinions, making judgments, and getting ideas. For instance, a major life change or life crisis may send you to the library or the Internet looking for information. You might talk to other people who have had similar experiences, create lists of questions to ask experts in the field, and then make decisions about what path you will follow. Often, this thinking brain is engaged first, leaving the feeling brain to follow when all the decisions have been made.

Early in her group experience, Jackie seemed to be engaging her thinking brain in the process of understanding Richard's illness—she needed answers to questions on treatments, side effects, doctors, and so forth. But as she became more comfortable with the group process, she started dealing with the feeling side of the situation. How could she communicate with family and friends? How could she and Richard gain strength through spirituality?

Feelings are your gut reactions to what has happened— your intuitive sense of what this means to you personally. Most feelings are expressed (or repressed) through one of the four basic emotions: glad, sad, mad, or scared. In group situations, the easiest emotion to express openly is being glad. We can all celebrate with others when their situation looks positive. But when people are sad (depressed), mad (angry), or scared (filled with fear), open disclosure becomes more difficult.

> Always remember to forget the things that
> made you sad,
> But never forget to remember the things that
> made you glad.
>
> —ELBERT HUBBARD

TELLING IT LIKE IT IS—HONESTLY!

You gain strength, courage, and confidence by every
experience in which you really stop to look fear in
the face.

—ELEANOR ROOSEVELT

Even in a fully developed, trusting group situation, full disclosure of our deepest emotions can be a daunting act of courage.
Honestly admitting to feelings of anger, resentment, fear, and
powerlessness when facing some of life's most serious challenges is a frightening process. Most people would choose to
sidestep that process and say nothing. But feelings are energy,
and denying feelings can distort behavior and judgment, ob-
scure perceptions, and cripple relationships. When we sidestep
the process of exposing our feelings, we block emotions.
When we block emotions, we block our ability to know and to
be sensitive to ourselves and others. As a result, our needs are
not met, and positive energy turns into distress and defensive-
ness. Instead of accepting, cherishing, and getting closer to the
ones we love, emotional distance causes us to judge, criticize,
withdraw, and become hostile.

Regardless of the life crisis—illness, death, physical abuse,
chemical dependency, loss of dreams—people will undoubtedly experience several common emotions when they react to
that crisis. How people respond to these emotions and share
them with friends and loved ones can have a profound effect
on the quality of those personal relationships. Honest communication is the key. And the issues that seem *most difficult*
to discuss are usually the ones needing the most attention.
Speaking honestly opens the door for growth.

UNDERSTANDING OUR EMOTIONS
AM I THE ONLY ONE WHO FEELS LIKE THIS?

Nothing in life is to be feared. It is only to be understood.

—MADAM CURIE

Sheri was understandably uncomfortable and afraid to talk about her innermost feelings surrounding Randy's illness when they were in the group together. She did not want to hurt him, and she knew that her darkest thoughts and fears would do just that. This is a common concern when groups are made up of both the people experiencing a loss personally *and* the family and the friends who are there to support them. Human nature makes people want to protect others and spare them any additional pain. And yet, putting up a good front—hiding behind a facade—can be draining and isolating. People need to find a way to vent these honest feelings and to learn that they are not alone in what they are experiencing.

For this reason, a large group might split into two for some meetings, giving the supportive people an opportunity to spend time together discussing these common emotions. At one particular session, Sheri and Jackie took part in such a discussion with several other group members who attend in support of a loved one. The emotions they discussed represented some universal feelings experienced by people going through a life change or life crisis.

Denial

Denial has been called nature's natural anesthetic and is a conditioned response to a situation that threatens to cause us great and immediate pain. Philip Slater, in the *Pursuit of Loneliness,* called it the toilet assumption—the notion that unwanted matter or difficulties would disappear if removed from our field of vision. "I don't believe it" is the conditioned response.

Early in Randy's diagnosis, Sheri admits that they both were in denial regarding its seriousness. "First, the doctors didn't really call it cancer, so we could deny that's what it really was," says Sheri. "We were convinced that the surgery would fix Randy and life would go on."

Now, almost five years later, Sheri fully understands the seriousness of Randy's condition. "I am seeing, through other group members, how denial can happen. I am trying to be realistic but often do not share in front of the group because Randy is usually there. I am starting to realize more and more what we are dealing with after seeing two close friends from group lose their spouses. It puts everything more in perspective."

Yet Sheri believes Randy is still denying the reality of it. Tonight she reports that Randy has become involved with a homeopathic practitioner who is promoting diet, nutrition, and supplements to "make Randy's cancer better." The practitioner stops short of calling it a cure, but Sheri is distressed by the disruption to the family. "He wants us all to eat the foods that Randy eats, and that's hard with young children," said Sheri. The group encouraged Sheri to continue feeding the children the usual foods, regardless of what Randy was doing. But Sheri's biggest concern again centers on denial. Is Randy using this as another way to deny what is really happening? Is he refusing to talk about the possibility of death because he is denying that it could happen?

Probably not, says Nancy, my cofacilitator who spent time that evening with Randy and the other people in the group who are living with cancer. Although Randy claimed that he was feeling better and that he believed the homeopathic remedies could help his cancer, he did not deny that his cancer had progressed to a nontreatable stage. With tears in his eyes, Randy clearly understood what was happening to him. His reticence to talk openly with Sheri was probably to protect her—the same reason she didn't want to speak openly in front of him. Nancy also stressed that, regardless of how *we* may want someone to respond, quite often their response may be just the opposite. Perfect communication just isn't going to happen. It might be just as important for Randy and Sheri to accept that they are both facing this situation in very different ways. And that is normal.

Would it help Randy and Sheri to be honest with one another about how they are truly feeling? Probably. Will it change the situation? No, but it might show that in real lives, terror and doubt keep daily company with hope and courage. It would show that Randy and Sheri are a normal family dealing with a difficult illness. They are experiencing a sometimes surreal existence where children act out and grownups fall into bed exhausted from too much stress. Sheri feels guilty for wanting time to herself. Randy is fearful of becoming dependent and a burden to those he loves. They both are terrified of losing one another. To open up to these emotions may allow them to share their life together in a deeper, more meaningful way.

Exposure of deep emotions is risky, but if we cling to a facade, to something that is not true, we deny ourselves the opportunity to bring about change. There is value for both Randy and Sheri—for all the group members—if they can look directly at their pain and not deny its existence.

Fear

Do the things you fear, and the death of fear is certain.

—RALPH WALDO EMERSON

Dorothy Bernard once defined *courage* as "fear that has said its prayers." Facing fear is the first step in conquering its power. Pretending it is not there is like not acknowledging the elephant sitting on the coffee table in the center of your living room. You know it's there, so talk about it. Fear increases in intensity in direct proportion to the length of time it takes you to confront it. And fear will take up as much of your life as you allow.

For Jackie, fear was mainly of the unknown. "I dealt with that by researching the disease as best I could—through the Internet, reading material, and the information gained at support group." Sheri found fear the most difficult emotion to share. "I always get emotional and cry. Mostly, I'm afraid of what's ahead, after seeing others in the group lose loved ones. I am young with three children and am scared to death."

Sister Arne's fear never seems to leave, especially after being diagnosed with a recurrence. "I've expressed this in support group, and just by saying it, I felt hope and received encouragement. Others have had similar fears and have learned to cope."

People gathered together for group support fear many things—the unknown, pain, helplessness and increased dependency on others, and loss of control. People who are accustomed to doing for others fear the burden of imposing their wants and needs on others. Many times, group members have had the expression of fears cut short by friends and family members trying to protect themselves from the pain of those fears. The supportive group environment helps people face their fears. In doing so, those fears don't seem quite so overwhelming, and group members feel closer to one another through their honest communication.

Anger/Resentment/Guilt

Anger is a short madness.

—HORACE

For all sad words of tongue or pen,
The saddest are these: "It might have been."

—JOHN GREENLEAF WHITTIER

How can this be happening to me? It isn't fair. Why me? Why now? People are angry at the life change or the crisis that is causing them pain and distress. And the expression of that anger can have peculiar overtones and can occur in very unexpected ways. Anger can be a mask to cover other more vulnerable feelings like sadness and fear. Or anger might surface as resentment and then quickly be followed by guilt. In the initial stages of a life crisis, panic shows itself in the disguise of anger.

Many people select a person or an institution on whom to vent their anger when reeling with pain. For Sheri, and for many people with cancer, it was the doctors. "We are frustrated with their knowledge about the disease and their inability to adequately share that with us," she said. "Most of us feel angry there is no cure." Said Jackie, "Anger flared up in various forms and at various times. We were angry at the disease, at each other, between Richard and our daughter, and among family members. Anger is not so much an issue once you are finally able to accept what is happening and try to deal with it best you can. We came to realize that we needed to make peace in order to make the best of our remaining time together."

When meeting alone together, friends and family members who are supporting individuals in crisis often admit to anger and resentment. Sheri feels guilty that she is resentful of Randy's inability to help her with the family. She feels guilty when she wants to leave all of them home and grab a few moments of peace by herself. "How can I justify getting angry with someone who is sick?" is a commonly expressed frustration coming from members of this group. They feel they must put all their needs on hold to satisfy the needs of the person who is sick. And if they don't, they end up feeling guilty. The group reminds Sheri that, although it is not unusual to feel guilty and blame yourself, most of the time the blame is undeserved. It's important for caregivers to understand that they are doing the best they can, given their circumstances. No one can expect more than that.

Marge and Ed joined the group when Ed's bladder cancer was discovered several years ago. After surgery for lung cancer last year, Ed recently experienced a recurrence and is undergoing chemotherapy. At 81, he remains active and lighthearted through it all, the "joker" in our group. When the group meets together, Ed never complains. His principal delight is drawing a laugh from the crowd.

In her private moments with the smaller subgroup, Marge looks at his lighthearted attitude a little differently. She admits to a certain resentment that Ed can be the life of the party in the group environment but not quite so cheery at home. And she sometimes gets angry when they always end up doing exactly what Ed wants to do. "Yesterday, I said I wanted to go to a department store to buy a pair of pants," Marge said. "Ed decided we should go to the hardware store first—on the way. By the time we had spent a half hour at the hardware store, Ed was tired, and we went home." The group encouraged Marge to find ways to get *both* of their needs met. Next time, she could drop him off at the hardware store before driving to the department store herself.

Anger we feel toward the person who is in pain is difficult to admit. But when the group lets us know that these feelings are natural and that we are not cold, unfeeling monsters, it seems easier to get past the anger and to find workable solutions. Similarly, the group can help the individual turn feelings of guilt, which are destructive and intent on self-blame, into feelings of remorse and sadness for "what might have been." Remember that the happiest people don't *have* the best of everything—they just *make* the best of everything.

Group members can learn from one another how to take responsibility for their own lives. By reminding one another that life is not fair, that people are not always reasonable, and that each person is responsible for his or her own feelings, group members gain the perspective and the strength to manage their own situations.

SELF-ESTEEM THROUGH SELF-AWARENESS

The psychic task which a person can and must set for himself is not to feel secure, but to be able to tolerate insecurity.

—ERICH FROMM

Being together with other people—hearing their stories, watching their coping styles—provides a mirror in which we can reflect on our own situation, which heightens our self-awareness and lessens our insecurities. Before joining the group, people may have felt incapable of the challenges being presented as a result of this new life crisis. They were uncertain of their roles and how they would accomplish the necessary tasks accompanying those roles. Being a part of a new community of kindred souls fosters personal growth by increasing each person's capacity to satisfy the requirements of the new roles they are being asked to play.

When we see others coping well in the face of a similar situation, it gives us an extra boost and reminds us that we are capable of similar coping abilities. We learn those new roles by interacting with people who are already playing those parts. By watching others in the process of learning, we see which methods succeed and which ones fail.

Not only did Sheri benefit from Jackie's physical support—taking care of the children, driving her to group, and so on—but she was able to use Jackie as a role model for how to behave as a supportive spouse. Jackie had been through it and had survived. Sheri's coping abilities were enhanced just knowing that others have walked the same path without completely losing their minds or giving up.

By the time the two smaller groups reconvened, the faces of the group members were noticeably less stressed. Their situations hadn't changed, but their attitudes about those situations had lightened. They had expressed their fears, angers, resentments, and concerns. The group had nurtured itself by taking one another seriously. They had listened, accepted, empathized, and supported one another. Without realizing it, each person had received a small intravenous injection of self-esteem.

PHASE 2—IN SEARCH OF SAFETY

> We cannot find reality simply by remaining with ourselves or making ourselves the goal. Paradoxically, we only know ourselves when we know ourselves in responding to others.
>
> —MAURICE FRIEDMAN

At each meeting, groups move closer to autonomy. Somewhere between being strangers and being members of a fully integrated group, individuals must learn how to work together. The rose-colored glasses that people wore as they were getting to know one another become more clear as the group matures. People begin to recognize one another's emotional holes and character flaws. As honest experiences and emotions are exposed and discussed, the group soon realizes that they are not always going to agree on important issues. One person may believe in homeopathic remedies. The next one may be adamantly opposed to such remedies, calling them quackery. They must learn how to express their differences—agree to disagree—without disrupting the value they derive from being part of the group.

As trust builds, group members learn to assert themselves as individuals and to differentiate their needs from the needs of the others in the group. People should be encouraged to say who they are and to ask for what they want, without fear of being put down or ostracized. Phase 2 is similar to adolescence or to the rebellious nature of teenagers on their way to the stable maturity of adulthood. Along the way, adolescents assert themselves and rebel as they struggle to find their independence within the structure of a community.

If the group provides safe haven during this period of stretching and if members are able to develop and assert their independence and individuality, the group will benefit and will grow into the deeper, trusting Phase 3 that follows. When open, honest communication is encouraged, and when each person acknowledges both individual and group needs, the group has a good chance of remaining viable and successful.

LEARNING TO LISTEN

To listen is to receive.

—ELIE WIESEL

At each meeting, we begin by informally taking roll and inquiring about any absences. Often, individual group members have talked to one another over the previous week and can report on activities of individuals who are not present. As groups develop, members do worry when people are missing from several meetings. Part of the structure could be to keep track of members' scheduled trips, doctor's appointments, treatment schedules, and so forth, so you can anticipate absences.

During the time when we are checking in with each person—listening to members share their victories and their fears—we try to develop a common theme for discussion. Rather than trying to predetermine a topic, it seems to be more productive to listen carefully to what is being said and let a theme evolve from the group's interests on that particular day. Major themes in groups that are dealing with a life change or life crisis seem to revolve around emotional topics like those mentioned earlier in this chapter. Many are struggling with the ways that the change in their life has affected their relationships with family and friends, communication problems, fear and anxiety, and balancing their needs against the needs of others.

Everyone yearns to be listened to. When we genuinely listen to another person, we are giving them the gift of our time and our respect. Yet, although listening is probably the most important component of effective groups, it is also the most difficult and neglected talent, by both facilitators and group members. We all know how to talk. But *two* parties are involved in any communication. And when someone else is talking, most of us would rather be thinking about ourselves and what we're going to say next. Instead, we should be listening—focusing on the person who is talking, not ourselves. Unless we learn to practice the skills necessary for effective listening, communication can be distorted.

Honest communication is a key ingredient to the success of support groups. For this reason, facilitators and members need to work at minimizing the distortion in that communication. This involves listening for *meaning* as well as *content* when people are sharing. Group process is enhanced by leadership that promotes deeper understanding and encourages further exploration. By practicing the following listening skills, every group member will enhance the value of the group's sharing time.

> Good listening is when we hear it all in balance, the little words and big words, the common and the uncommon.
>
> —EVELYN OPPENHEIMER

Focus on the Speaker

Focusing on the speaker means that you are "with" that person, physically, mentally, and emotionally. Turn your body toward the speaker, block out any sight or sound diversions, and give that person your full concentration. Make eye contact that seems comfortable for the other person. Make a conscious effort to keep your eyes and ears open, and your mouth shut.

As you listen, occasionally nod your head or add a few words, such as "I see" or "uh-huh" just to let the speaker know you are still listening. This shows your interest and gives the speaker encouragement to continue. If the speaker appears to be rambling, repeating, or going in an unrelated direction, try to redirect the thoughts back to the original thought.

Listen without Judging

Nonjudgmental acceptance is the cornerstone of any group philosophy and is also an important component of listening. Listening without judging provides safe haven. People who feel they are not being judged or labeled naturally feel safe and accepted. Through appropriate listening, group members can learn to respect one another, even if they don't agree with one another. Once this trust is established, members are more likely to share their innermost concerns and feelings. Good listeners leave their own personal value systems out of the equation.

Listen for Feelings

When you focus and pay close attention, you will hear more than the speaker's words. You will watch their body language and see their facial expression. You will hear the tone of voice and the amount of emotion in that tone. When you combine all these elements, you begin to get a complete picture of what that person is feeling as they speak.

Try to see the world through the speaker's eyes. Try to imagine yourself in that person's place. If you truly have been there, you can *empathize* and respond from your gut. If you have not been there but can understand what the person is saying and are concerned, then you can *sympathize*.

Do a mental tally, and add up the negative versus positive feelings being voiced. Does this person look distressed, even though the words don't say so? If you feel a dissonance between what is being said and the person's nonverbal communication, try to draw out the reasons for this difference.

Remember that feelings aren't right or wrong—they just are. People need to feel safe sharing their feelings without fear of retribution.

Listen with Understanding

When people are sharing honest feelings, they want to believe you understand. You can show you do by periodically checking out what you are hearing. When you respond, use words that include both the *content* of what you heard and the *feelings* expressed. Marge's story of wanting to go to a department store but ending up at a hardware store would be a common (almost humorous) story under normal circumstances. But as Marge told the story, her intensity as she spoke and her serious tone of voice divulged her own emotional reactions to the content of the story. A responsive statement that shows understanding and probes further might be: "That story sounds like something that has happened to all of us, Marge, but it seems like it meant more to you. What were you thinking when this all happened?"

When the speaker knows you were listening, that person is encouraged to elaborate further and to go deeper for the emotional meaning of what he or she has said.

Listen for What Is Important

Group members often take long, circuitous paths before arriving at that all-important destination—the point of the story. People wander and drift as they talk, and one thing leads to another. Either a leader or another group member can make this observation and steer the speaker back on track. Try to remember where the person started out—this is often a key to where they were trying to go. If they drift too far from that starting point, find ways to redirect the conversation back to the beginning. Keeping speakers "on task" benefits the whole group by eliminating confusion and frustration.

Listen—To Show You Care

The most important reason why we listen to people carefully is that we care about them and their feelings. We know that the greatest gift we can give them is our time, our acceptance, and our encouragement. Sometimes it takes a personal story to bring home the damage that can be done when the value of listening is not taken seriously.

During the writing of this portion of the book, our Affirming Life group had an important and moving discussion related to the fine art of listening. For the past year, Pat had been in a very healthy remission from a breast cancer recurrence. But after a serious bout with the flu this past winter, she had been having trouble regaining her strength. Lately, she has been filled with anxiety. Her feelings remind her of how anxious and disoriented she was when her breast cancer recurred, for the second time, in 1997. The group encouraged her to see her primary doctor regarding the anxiety.

On this day she reported the very disquieting results from that visit. "The doctor didn't look at me when I was telling him my symptoms. Instead, he kept paging through my chart while I was talking. He kept mumbling about 1993 and 1997 and the details surrounding my breast cancer. He was not listening at all to the reason I was there that day—my anxiety and weak stomach after being sick with the flu. Finally, he said something about breast cancer spreading to the stomach, and maybe I should have a CAT scan."

This doctor broke all the rules laid out in this chapter. He did not focus on Pat and give her his undivided attention. He did not listen for feelings. He responded by judging the situation instead of trying to understand what Pat was saying. He made false and erroneous assumptions. Finally, he did not focus on what was important that day.

By not listening, this doctor caused Pat more anxiety instead of helping her cope with her situation. She walked out of his office more upset and confused than when she arrived.

Barriers to Good Listening

Well-placed road signs help us avoid accidents on the road. In the same way, we can prevent accidents in communication by knowing what to look for. The following six negative behaviors will not only affect your listening skills but will also inhibit the group's ability to communicate effectively. Watch for them in yourself, and caution group members against using them as well. These same barriers are covered in Discussion Guide #4 at the end of this chapter.

Moralizing "You should," "You shouldn't," "You must" are all moralizing phrases that bring shame on the other person while exalting your status. Stop yourself from speaking before you make judgments.

Downplaying "Don't worry about it, everything will be fine." This kind of downplaying is heard often by cancer survivors. Although these are usually well-intentioned comments, they actually are telling the speaker that you are not interested in what they are saying and that what they are feeling is not important.

Advising "Here's what I did . . ." How often have you listened to someone's problem and immediately jumped in with *your* solution? Remember that when people are sharing, they are not looking for your solutions. They are trying to better understand their own situation before making their own decisions. Help them out by withholding your advice.

Lecturing "I think I know what's best for you." Parents are experts at lecturing. Just ask our children. Lecturing talks down to the other person, insinuating that they matter less and know less than you. Groups meet to provide support, not assert superiority.

Partiality We all have biases or preferences of thinking. A common example of letting this partiality get out of control is "doctor bashing." We have a ground rule disallowing this practice. Each group member should be aware of his or her own biases and be sure not to let those biases interfere with his or her acceptance of others in the group.

Inappropriate Humor As discussed previously, appropriate humor can lighten the group. When someone has shared a situation or a feeling that is personal or significant, ill-timed or misused humor could be considered abusive.

Mastering and practicing the fine art of listening helps the group progress to the next level. When you listen because you care, your genuineness and sincerity shine through and are reflected back in the faces of every group member.

> Unless you listen, you can't know anybody. Oh, you will know facts and what is in the newspapers and all of history, perhaps, but you will not know one single person. You know, I have come to think listening is love, that's what it really is.
>
> —BRENDA UELAND

The Fine Art of Storytelling

In the Introduction of this book, you met four people whose lives were in crisis. One of them was Joan, a former co-worker of mine who tragically lost her 12-year-old daughter when they were both struck by lightning. In the early months after the accident, many of Joan's friends and co-workers felt helpless. They wanted to say or do things, but they didn't know what. "People brought meals every night for months," Joan remembers. "Finally, when my freezer was stuffed to overflowing with leftovers, I had to stop them." What Joan needed the most from these people was for them to listen to her tell her story—again and again and again.

The Power of Stories

> At last the secret is out, as it always must come
>   in the end;
> The delicious story is ripe to tell to the intimate
>   friend;
> Over the tea cups and in the square the tongue
>   has its desire;
> Still waters run deep, my dear, there's never
>   smoke without fire.

—W. H. Auden

In the past, people sat around the table after a meal and talked. Women got together over coffee in their homes while men gathered around a table at the main street café. Congregations gathered in fellowship hall after services. Folks sat on the front porch and yelled out to passing neighbors. Stories were shared daily in a variety of ways.

But today, in our hurry-up world, filled with cell phones, beepers, e-mail, and the Internet, has storytelling become a fossil like upright typewriters and dial phones? Hopefully not, because the telling of stories is what brings a unique richness to a small community of people. Stories are the backdrop against which we come to truly know the personality of another person and what is important to them.

Stories of ordinary experiences are the connective tissue that binds groups together as well. No one is excluded from the discussion, because each of us has a story to tell. And through the telling of our personal stories, we can retain our individuality, while at the same time finding commonalities among our fellow group members.

Why Tell Our Stories?

Our stories make us unique. As we put into words the various elements of our lives that have been meaningful, a pattern emerges of who we are. We become our stories by telling and retelling them. Through our stories, not only are other people getting to know us, but we are learning more about ourselves— who and what contributed to making us what we are today.

Our stories help with relationships and community. In the early stages of group development, personal stories help people connect in a very personal way. The development of Jackie and Sheri's relationship was based on their stories and how they related those stories to the group. When the group has been together longer, they become a source for stories about themselves as a community. Our group often shares the story of attending a funeral of a group member together. At the time, Randy was in a wheel chair. Several members picked up that wheelchair (with Randy in it) and quickly whisked him up the long, steep stairway into the church. They retell this story over and over as a reminder to themselves of how much they mean to one another.

Our stories inspire and connect us with the humanness of others. Sheri gets plenty of advice from others on how to manage her life in the face of Randy's illness. But advice normally does not inspire us. Listening to Jackie talk about her experience and how she handled each stage of Richard's illness is what inspires Sheri. Through Jackie, Sheri has hope that whatever the future holds, she can manage the situation. We are inspired by the events that have shaped real people's lives, not by unsolicited advice. When we hear others tell stories of failure and success, sorrow and joy, gifts and losses, we truly understand our collective humanity and are inspired to gain a fresh perspective and to forgive our own shortcomings.

Our stories connect us with our feelings. As we tell our story, we vent feelings that must come out. By expressing the feelings, the teller can detach from them and gain a better insight into the situation. Marge's story of the trip to the hardware store was more than just a story. It allowed her to express feelings of resentment about which she had never talked before. (An interesting note is that Marge pulled me aside the next week to tell me that since the last meeting, she had gotten to the store for the pants all on her own. She seemed pretty proud. We do find solutions once we air our problems.)

Our stories help us understand our truth. The complexity of life today makes it more and more difficult to answer even the most basic questions about the nature of human existence. Science, metaphysics, philosophy, and theology all have their own theories. But perhaps our stories are the real answer to fundamental questions about the way life is. Our stories explain how we arrived here, where we were before, and what the differences are. Harvard psychologist Jerome Bruner says that this kind of self-discovery actually allows us to reconstruct ourselves. Not only do we remember our past, but we get a glimpse of how our past changed us. This revelation can then guide our behavior in the present and help us set our moral compass for the future. As Soren Kierkegaard said,

"Life can only be understood backwards; but it must be lived forwards."

Through structure, active listening, and storytelling, groups develop trust and start to build deeper relationships. For more information on specific group-building tips, see Chapter Seven.

Discussion Guide #3
Getting in Touch with Our Emotions

The emotional environment we create within our bodies can activate mechanisms of either destruction or repair.

BACKGROUND MATERIAL

Emotional disclosure is a large part of group dynamics. As individuals work through their situations by sharing with others, feelings that may have been withheld or misunderstood now come to the surface. Some people cry for the first time when they start talking in the group. Others might be shocked to hear a family member or a friend express anger or resentment.

Although it feels like people are risking everything by admitting their real feelings, honest emotional disclosure is necessary if people are going to grow and learn. The treatment of emotional issues is just as important as treating physical issues.

> Not everything that is faced can be changed. But nothing can be changed until it is faced.
>
> —JAMES BALDWIN

DISCUSSION/GROUP EXERCISE

Personalize this meeting by using emotions that the group seems to be experiencing. This same exercise can be used with other emotions such as guilt, denial, anxiety, or grief.

List the following emotions on a chalkboard or overhead projector, and elicit response and discussion from group members.

Anger and Fear

Anger and fear are common reactions to a life-changing event. Why link them together? Because although you may *feel* angry, that feeling is sometimes a mask for the fear that lies just below the surface. The reasons for anger and fear are varied. In this group experience, it is important that individuals admit to their fear and anger, understand that they are common and acceptable emotions, and learn how to share them with others. The task of the discussion is learning how to find ways to channel that anger without harming yourself or others.

- Name things, situations, or occurrences that make you angry.
- What do you believe causes the anger?
- What are some creative ways you have learned to handle the anger?
- Brainstorm among group members and list responses.

Sadness/Depression

Depression or mental dysfunction occurs frequently and is dependent on numerous factors, including the severity of the situation, previous coping patterns, economic resources, availability of a support system, and availability of good medical care. The task of the discussion is to help group members identify the factors that may be causing the depression and to develop individualized plans to counteract these factors.

- Name some factors that you believe have caused your sadness or your depression.
- What are some creative things you can do to bring joy back to your life?
- Brainstorm among group members and list responses.

Fatigue

Many people expect fatigue in times of physical or emotional crisis. The task of this discussion is to help group members try to identify causes of fatigue (stress, insomnia, medications, etc.) and to help them learn healthy ways to counteract fatigue—or to accept it as part of the healing process.

- Name some factors that you believe are causing your fatigue.
- Are you physically tired, or are you perhaps emotionally or spiritually tired?
- How are you experiencing fatigue (having difficulty making body move or making words come out right; can't think; having emotional outbursts; trouble staying awake)?
- What creative ways do you use to combat fatigue?
- Brainstorm among group members and list responses.

SUMMARY

Conclude the discussion by affirming that feelings aren't right or wrong, they just are. All of the above emotions discussed are normal and to be expected. Encourage group members to share their honest emotions with one another and with family members and friends.

Discussion Guide #4
Learning How to Listen

Hear the other side.

BACKGROUND INFORMATION

Listening is as important to communication as speaking. Until the recipient "gets the message," communication is incomplete. A good exercise is to simply listen to someone else, without reacting or responding. It's difficult! We all are anxious to be heard, but active listening takes practice and discipline.

GROUP EXERCISE

Divide your group into pairs. In each pair, one person will listen while the other tells about a person who has been a big influence or has been very important in his or her life. Allow five minutes for the telling of the story. Then ask the listener to share what was heard. If time permits, have them reverse roles and do the exercise again.

When the exercise is complete, have the group get back together to evaluate what happened. Use the following questions to assess the experience, and then come to some conclusions on what constitutes effective listening.

1. Did you feel that your partner was listening to you? Why or why not?

2. What signals did your partner give that made you feel that he or she was listening (or not listening)?
3. Do you believe your partner heard your feelings as well as your words? Why?
4. Did your partner use words or body language that signified genuine listening? What were they?
5. What is the most important lesson you learned from this exercise?

SUMMARY

Learning to listen means learning to close your mouth and open your ears. It means learning to concentrate not only on *what* is being said, but on *how* it is being said. It means listening for words, tone of voice, rate of speech, attitude, body language, and missing pieces.

Discussion Guide #5
Turning Weaknesses into Strengths

An optimist is one who makes the best of conditions,
after making the conditions the best possible.

BACKGROUND MATERIAL

All human situations are powerfully influenced by the individual's *perception* of the situation. Group members cannot change the situation in which they find themselves, but they can change how they think about it. People who study the effects of the mind on healing are learning that attitude is very important to healing. Unresolved conflict, internalized anger, and fear can combine to suppress the immune system. Stress can make people sick, while dealing openly with emotions can contribute to good health.

During this group exercise, remember that emotions aren't right or wrong, they just are. Group members should be encouraged to share feelings and emotions. The purpose of the exercise is to find positive ways to look at what may be perceived as negative events.

GROUP EXERCISE

Use the following questions as discussion guides, and write them on a chalkboard, flip chart, or overhead projector. Encourage the group to discuss a variety of life-affirming activities that can turn weaknesses into strengths.

- Under what conditions and in what environment do you feel most optimistic about your ability to deal with your life situation? What does that tell you about how you could modify your day-to-day activities to make certain you are capitalizing on that environment?
- What activities, groups, or individuals help you affirm your self-worth?
- Reflect back to the time when you were most distressed about your life situation. Now reflect back and remember any positive changes that have taken place during this period of crisis and/or change in your life. What progress have you made? Give yourself credit!
- What do you perceive as your greatest weakness? Your greatest strength? How can you apply that strength to its best advantage to help you overcome the weakness?

SUMMARY

Group members can turn weaknesses into strengths by honestly assessing their progress and by challenging themselves to set realistic goals for reshaping their lives. Even a small step forward boosts self-worth and gives people the impetus to try a little harder for that next step.

Chapter Four
Finding Your Spiritual Core

With God, all things are possible.

—St. Matthew 19:26

Dennis went into Alcoholics Anonymous kicking and screaming. "It's not hard for me to remember what it was like, even though it was 23 years ago, because I repeat the story at almost every meeting," he says. "As a drinking alcoholic, I had been through treatment six times, had been taken to a variety of AA meetings, but (as is true with most of us) nothing had penetrated very much. To sum it up, I wasn't a good candidate for success."

Then Dennis met three men who changed his life—his sponsors. They were adamant about picking him up and getting him to meetings. In the small Midwestern town of 30,000, those meetings took place every night. And Dennis went every night, because his sponsors insisted. Most nights he went drunk. "I hated going. It made me nervous, so I ended up drinking more," Dennis remembers. "After each meeting, when they brought me home, invariably I asked them to not pick me up for another meeting." But the next night, they were at his door again.

They would continue to ask, "Do you have the desire to quit drinking?" And Dennis would always say yes, but qualify it with a firm belief that he could never quit. He was heartless and hopeless. "I had quit drinking hundreds of times, and it never worked," he says. "I had given up hope of ever succeeding."

But as the days and weeks wore on, Dennis's resistance was worn down by his sponsors' unswerving belief in him. Finally, one fateful day, he had his last drink. He went directly into chemical dependency treatment. And he has been sober ever since. "The group's unwillingness to give up on me in spite of all my resistance was something I had never seen before. I had been religious all my life—I had even been in the seminary. But I had never experienced spirituality in quite that way. My true faith started in AA."

UNDERSTANDING DEPRESSION

Despite the positive effects of a group experience, people enduring difficult life situations will have days when it seems as if they don't have the strength to go forward. Signs of depression creep in. But is it really *depression?* Because this word is so overused in our culture, sometimes it's hard to know when people are experiencing "the real thing." Feelings of sadness are to be expected when facing a life crisis, but this doesn't qualify as true depression. We all have down days; and usually, being down, being sad, means that we are missing what we have lost—a loved one, our health, a relationship. But in the natural order of things, this sadness leads to healing.

Severe clinical depression, on the other hand, is an illness demanding expert medical attention, and it is characterized by a complete lack of feeling. If you have depression, you don't care about anything. Eating habits may change—you either eat too much or not enough. Sleeping habits may change— you either sleep too much or not enough. You are unmotivated and lose interest in things that you formerly enjoyed.

You can't concentrate on a task. You may cry or lose your temper more often. You are feeling worthless and are highly self-critical. If you are living with a chronic illness, these signs of depression may be confused with symptoms of illness.

As the depression progresses and intensifies, however, the spiral of despondency and hopelessness worsens. You withdraw from friends, and a dark blanket of sorrow spreads itself over each day's events. You feel a sense of futility—that this pain will never leave you. Regardless of the joyousness of an event, you are unable to marshall a sense of joy for anything. At this point, it's time to talk to your doctor. If you don't, you run the risk of getting into a pattern of behavior in which the depression controls all your thoughts and actions. You may even begin thinking that suicide is the only way out.

Clinical depression afflicts more than 17 million people in the United States each year. Many see it as a weakness or a character flaw and refuse to seek treatment. Instead, they choose to just tough it out. This decision could lead to months or years of torment. In fact, depression is a chemical imbalance in the brain that usually can be corrected with antidepressants.

New medications have made an enormous difference in the fight against depression. Once a person starts on a drug, however, it may take as long as two weeks to feel its effects. Full benefit from the medications takes six months to a year. In addition to medication, talk therapy can help people learn how to end self-defeating patterns and how to work through the issues that caused the depression. Exercise also helps, because exercise releases brain chemicals called endorphins—stimulants that help fight off depression. If you suspect you are depressed, contact a physician or a mental health professional for a consultation. Whether it's medication, therapy, or a combination of both, depression is treatable. If you suspect that someone in your group is clinically depressed, based on the symptoms he or she reports, you should suggest that the group leader talk with that person one-on-one about a referral to a mental health professional. Make sure that the signs and symptoms of clinical depression are discussed within your group setting.

The encouraging, supportive environment of a group has helped many people work through mild depression. Regular attendance at group meetings can put an end to the self-inflicted isolation that is often a symptom of depression. Words of encouragement and acceptance from others can put a hopeful spin on an otherwise dark situation. In addition, many people connect with a higher power for additional support and hope.

CONNECTING WITH A HIGHER POWER

Religion is not asking. It is a longing of the soul.

—GANDHI

It is only to the individual that a soul is given.

—ALBERT EINSTEIN

My soul is overwhelmed with sorrow to the point of death.

—MATTHEW 26:38

When people are caught up in sadness or mild depression, they may begin to give up on life and the day-to-day activities that have been keeping them in the mainstream. As they sink further and further, many begin soul searching—looking outside themselves for something to provide strength and guidance. This kind of searching represents a desire to connect with a "higher power," which is an integral part of AA's program.

If you ask Dennis about the spiritual aspect of Alcoholics Anonymous, he corrects the assumption made in the question—that spirituality is a *part* of AA. Rather, he sees spirituality at the core of AA. "Drinking is only the symptom of a spiritual disorder that affects us physically, mentally, and spiritually," he says. "When I declared to my sponsors that I was without hope—powerless over my drinking—they reminded me that I didn't have to do this alone. There was help in the form of a higher power."

Dennis admits that in the beginning—when all you want to do is clean up your act, pay your bills, go to meetings, and stay sober—thoughts about the significance of that higher power may be far from your mind. But as the group members go through the first 3 steps of a 12-step program, they begin to make the connection between their powerlessness and that gift of a higher power. Does this mean forcing religion on people who do not consider themselves religious? Dennis says no. "We don't tell people they need to go to church or believe in God," Dennis says. "But we do ask them to reflect on how successful they had been trying to go it alone—relying on their own free will to stay sober. Most have to admit they were failing."

Dennis goes on to say that each person's higher power is unique to that person. It may be the group. It may be God. It may be the Buddha. "Just so long as you recognize that help comes in the form of a higher power—that it's not *you, the person*." The spiritual growth that takes place in AA happens as a consequence of being involved over the long haul. Early in membership, people often balk at the third step, which is turning their will and their lives over to that higher power. But they usually make the spiritual connection between their inability to handle alcohol alone and the success they achieve within AA. What made the difference? Realizing that human power alone could not relieve their suffering. Seeking a higher power made the difference. And continued group attendance reminds them over and over again of the wisdom of their decision.

Today, when someone asks Dennis how he got through a difficult life situation without drinking, he says: "I didn't—God got me through." To him, this is not a profound spiritual concept. It's survival.

Dennis's experience with AA appears to be universal within this organization. That does not mean that all groups approach spirituality in the same way. It is safe to say, however, that a sense of the spiritual becomes a part of almost every group experience. How that spirituality is identified becomes very unique to each group.

WHY ME, LORD?

How can great wisdom care so little about the torments of the innocent creatures? This question, which began to agonize me when I was six or seven years old, still haunts me today. I still cannot accept the ruthlessness of nature, God, the Absolute. . . . How can a merciful God allow all this to happen and keep silent?

—ISAAC B. SINGER

People confronted with a life crisis often wrestle with the higher power in their lives by asking the big question: Why me? Some accept the limits of human knowledge and are satisfied with a simplistic answer: Why not you? But others begin to believe that God is punishing them for something they have done wrong. They may feel abandoned by their God and confused and resentful at how they have been treated. After all, they had followed all the rules, gone to church, and lived a pious life, only to be rewarded with this cruel blow.

Unfortunately, death, illness, broken relationships, and accidents happen to all of us—the pure and the evil. Chemical dependency is a result of a chemical and physical imbalance. Just because bad things happen to good people does not mean that God is punishing us. It means that God has placed us in a human world, and just being human is risky business. Life is often not very fair, and we must endure hard times.

In the face of this cruel reality, many people find hope by assigning meaning to their suffering. This search for meaning becomes that person's spiritual journey, and each one is unique. In his famous book, *Man's Search for Meaning*, Viktor Frankl states that "what matters is not the meaning of life in general, but rather the specific meaning of a person's life at a given moment." In the end, life ultimately means "taking the responsibility to find the right answer to its problems and to fulfill the tasks which it constantly sets for each individual." Each group member's individual burdens are very different, even though members come to the group with a common problem. What nourishes one person's soul may be totally in-effective for another. But generally, people with a strong spirit and a true belief understand that there is a place in the human experience for suffering. Each individual's personal spiritual journey helps that person transcend the pain and the loss and turn them into something meaningful.

Joan thought she had been religious all her life. She had grown up attending a Lutheran church, had gone to Sunday school, memorized the catechism, and faithfully took her own children to church. In the days and weeks following the light-ning strike and her daughter Jen's death on Minnesota's re-mote Gunflint Trail, Joan struggled to understand why. Why would a loving God take a 12-year-old child? She and her hus-band went to their pastor for help. They were both surprised to learn that he didn't know what to do for them. Thankfully, he sent them to Compassionate Friends, a support group for parents who had lost children.

"Before I went, I thought we were the only ones on the planet who knew the pain—that no one in the world could possibly fathom what we were going through," she remem-bers. "But what we realized is that all the parents in the room understood. Although their stories were different, their pain was the same. It helped because we could tell others what hap-pened, again and again. Each time, as I cried and told the story, I began to get more control of the situation."

Group support gave Joan permission to celebrate Jen's life in whatever way she chose. The family placed her picture on the gravestone and covered it with a clear dome. Now, rain or snow, they can see her smiling face when they visit. Jen's siblings planted an evergreen tree near the grave, and they decorate the tree for every holiday. At Christmas, the tree is covered with brilliant red poinsettias. At Easter, brightly decorated Easter eggs adorn the branches. But the religious holidays only reminded Joan more of her unresolved conflict with her God. The unanswered question of "why" still gnawed at her heart. "Compassionate Friends helped us in many ways, but they couldn't help me satisfy the spiritual piece," says Joan. "I needed to look further."

For three months, she counseled with the Director of Spiritual Care at a health care organization. "He helped me just talk it out," she remembers. "We wrestled time and again with why a loving God would do this." It was during this time that Joan began meeting with a group of close friends and family who were also trying to make sense of Jen's death. They started a Bible study group to see if the Bible could help answer their questions. Thus began Joan's second group experience, all part of her personal spiritual journey to answer the question, why me, Lord?

"First, I needed to know where she was," Joan says. "I knew in my heart of hearts that she was in heaven. The last message she left on her whiteboard in her bedroom was a paraphrasing of Psalm 23: 'Even though I walk through darkness, your rod and staff will guide me every day.' It's still there. I haven't erased it."

Joan knew Jen was in heaven. "Now I needed to know how to get there, because I want to see my baby again," Joan continues. "As a Lutheran, I was raised to believe that we enter heaven by grace. As our group continued to read the Bible, it became more complicated than that. We came to understand that Jesus Christ died on the cross for our sins, and believing in him would give us eternal life."

Through her second group experience—a Bible study group—Joan changed from having religion to having a relationship with her God. "All those years of going to church and reading and memorizing had meant nothing to me," Joan says. "Now, my personal relationship with God has given me peace."

After Jen's death, Joan had been consumed with trying to understand why. Today she no longer agonizes over that question. "The why doesn't matter anymore," she says. And her eyes reflect her sense of reconciliation with the tragedy in her life. "'Some sweet day, we'll be together again,'" Joan says, repeating the words of a popular song that she and her husband listen to almost daily. "When we are together again—when I finally meet my God—the first place I'm going is to the answer booth. Then I'll find out why." Joan now believes that her personal relationship with God developed as a result of her daughter's death. Because of that newfound relationship, their family will someday be complete again. Somehow, that attaches meaning to her sorrow.

Joan found meaning in her suffering through a better understanding of God. Dennis credits the presence of a higher power for his 23 years of sobriety. Belief in a higher power and the effect it can have on your life is a powerful source of hope, for now and for the future.

SPIRITUALITY EQUALS CONNECTION, MEANING, AND HOPE

Connection

> To be closer to God, be closer to people.
>
> —KAHLIL GIBRAN

Spirituality has been defined as our deepest sense of belonging and connectedness to life. This connectedness to something or someone outside of ourselves strengthens our inner resources. Regardless of an individual's personal religious beliefs, belonging to a group often creates this kind of spiritual connection. This may take place because the ground rules for most groups of kindred souls stress nonjudgmental acceptance, encouragement, listening, trust, and forgiveness. These are the same values that foster the spiritual dimension in human relationships. Without even trying, group members sense that something sacred is taking place, even though no formal spiritual component is present.

Finding Meaning

The meaning of our existence is not invented by ourselves, but rather detected. What matters, therefore, is not the meaning of life in general, but rather the specific meaning of a person's life at a given moment.

—VIKTOR FRANKL

People also get in touch with their own spiritual dimension when they identify a meaning or a purpose in life. As Frankl stated, this does not signify the meaning of life in general, but a specific meaning at a given moment. Prior to Jen's death, Joan had not looked deeply at the meaning of life. But this tragedy forced Joan to look deep and to search for a way to make sense of something that was totally senseless. She found her answers by connecting with other people and by connecting with a personal God. In Minnesota, Patty Wetterling's life changed the day her son Jacob was kidnapped while riding his bike on a remote country road. Today, more than 10 years later, she continues to assign meaning to her son's kidnapping through her work to establish the Jacob Wetterling Foundation, which helps other parents work through the pain associated with kidnapping. Mothers Against Drunk Drivers (MADD) was established by a mother who lost a child to a drunk driver. You can probably think of many other examples of similar actions that assigned meaning to a tragedy.

Viktor Frankl believes that we discover meaning in one of three ways: (1) by doing a deed; (2) by experiencing a value; and (3) by suffering.

Obviously, most of the people profiled in this book have suffered. In his suffering, Dennis experienced an important value—that he did not have to do it alone. "My faith started in AA," he says. "It was the first time I really believed that I was not responsible to make sure the universe ran the way it was supposed to run. I finally learned I could get more done by letting go."

Having Hope

> Hope and hopelessness are both choices, so why not choose hope?
>
> —GREG ANDERSON

> Hope means to keep living amid desperation and to keep humming in the darkness.

The need for hope is another dimension of a person's spirituality. Although a well-functioning hope is always based in reality, its purpose is to guard against despair by repressing doubts and fears. The main difference between hope and denial is that hope transcends reality, whereas denial avoids reality.

Hope is not static; it changes as situations and circumstances change. Hope comes in many forms—hope for healing, hope for a good life in the future, hope for meaningful relationships, hope for caring and support, hope for a comfortable death. Support groups often become communities of hope. Group members consistently remind one another of the fact that there is always something to hope for. They share their own personal hopes and dreams and teach others by example.

Joan lives each day in the hope that the family will someday be reunited with Jen. Dennis lives in the hope of lifetime sobriety. Members of our Affirming Life group for women with recurrent cancer hope for a variety of things, all based on the progression of their illness. Donna hopes for a continued long remission. Sister Arne hopes for freedom from pain. Candy hopes to see her children grow up. One group member hopes that the time spent on an Alaskan cruise will be free of cancer symptoms. Hope gives us peace in the midst of turmoil and continued strength for the day.

The Journey of Faith

We shall not cease from exploration,
and the end of all our exploring
Will be to arrive where we started,
and know the place for the first time.

—T. S. Eliot

In his book *Sharing the Journey,* author Robert Wuthnow's surveys confirmed that group sharing contributes to the members' spiritual development. "Specifically, 61 percent of all group members say their faith or spirituality has been influenced by being involved in their group." His findings indicate that millions of people are on a journey in search of a spiritual life. Yet, in today's secular society, with its emphasis on speed, technology, and material wealth, instead of finding spiritual fulfillment, many people are drowning in their own excesses. It is not surprising that many find their spiritual life lacking and are feeling a need to embark on a spiritual journey. Because material wealth hasn't satisfied their longings, they are finally ready to admit that happiness comes from within. Perhaps only a spiritual journey can help them discover how to tap into that happiness. And a journey cannot be traveled alone. Pilgrims need other pilgrims. Being in the company of kindred souls provides guidance and support for the journey.

As group members come to trust one another and to learn from one another, they begin to feel like they are on the same spiritual journey. Through telling their stories and sharing with others, people disclose integral pieces of their inner world. This kind of disclosure helps individuals understand themselves better. When they disclose their deepest thoughts to another person, that disclosure demystifies the process. They then can step back and examine what they have said. This helps them to identify their strongest motivations and the things that strengthen the spirit.

Each person in a group has a unique way of expressing his or her spirit. As part of the honest sharing, acceptance, and unconditional love within the group, connections happen at a heart level. Boundaries fall away, and each person's individuality is absorbed into the group's collective soul. Each person becomes a part of something larger than himself or herself. Call it spirit, energy, consciousness, or love, something happens among kindred souls that is larger than life, deeper than human. This group spirit is a way of feeling God's presence and a good beginning for understanding the nature and the mystery of each person's spiritual dimension.

TRUSTING ENOUGH TO LET GO

God made Truth with many doors to welcome every believer who knocks on them.

—KAHLIL GIBRAN

Having the faith to let go and to trust in a higher power has a paradoxical effect. People end up feeling more in control. For the first time, Dennis realized that he didn't need to be in control because something greater than him was in charge. Faith implies trust. And because trust is one of the key components of a group of kindred souls, people learn to understand the power of faith. Faith is a simple acceptance of life as it comes our way. "Let go—let God" is a familiar phrase heard at group meetings. Through group interaction, people learn to trust that life is still good, even though bad things happen to good people.

Today, Dennis has a deepened faith and thoroughly trusts his God. "I know God cares about me and is involved in my life," he says. "I learned that I need to stay out of the driver's seat. At the first sign of self-will, I give it over to God, and things go much better."

THE POWER OF PRAYER

Ask, and it shall be given you; Seek and ye shall find; Knock and the door will be opened unto you.

—MATTHEW 7:7

When we pray, we don't change the world. We change ourselves.

—RACHEL NAOMI REMEN, M.D., *KITCHEN TABLE WISDOM*

Randolph Byrd, working out of the cardiac care unit at San Francisco General Hospital, researched the effect of prayer on about 400 of his patients. All were treated with routine standard care, but half of the patients (without their knowledge) also had various prayer groups praying for them. The difference in outcomes was striking. The prayed-for group experienced no cardiac arrests or need for ventilators. Twelve people in the other group either arrested or required some form of further treatment.

Larry Dossey in his book, *Healing Words: The Power of Prayer and the Practice of Medicine,* documents this story along with many others on the powerful effect of prayer. "Prayer says something incalculably important about who we are and what our destiny may be," says Dossey. He goes on to point out that the studies on prayer show no correlation between religious affiliation and the effects of prayer in the laboratory. The factors at work appear to be love, compassion, empathy, and deep caring. Groups of kindred souls, by their very nature, share these important factors. For this reason, the power of prayer within the confines of a group can be very powerful.

Groups help people stay in touch with their prayers. They remind one another of specific prayers that they believe have been answered. They feel nurtured and cared for when they know that others are praying for them. Rather than simply praying in a generic way, groups pray in very specific, meaningful ways for the good of one another. Such specialized prayers help the group members become closer, and they feel a closer relationship with their higher power, both individually and collectively. Margaret Poloma and George Gallup did a national study of prayer and found that "the most profound effects of prayer occur when a person goes beyond rote and ritualistic prayer and senses an intimacy with God." Groups who include prayer as part of their normal agenda sense this type of intimacy.

Dossey wrote about a group called Spindrift out of Salem, Oregon, who researched the effect of prayer on simple biological systems. Spindrift found that nondirected prayer (Thy will be done) was more effective than petitionary prayer (I pray that I will be cured of my cancer). Groups usually avoid petitionary prayer. In most cases, they pray for healing, for strength, or for resolution to a problem.

Dossey concludes, however, by suggesting that people should not get hung up on a formula. "It would be abuse of information to attempt to prescribe how one should pray, image, or visualize," he said in an interview with Daniel Redwood. "You don't have to follow what any authority says. Do what's right for you. Turn inward and turn upward."

May we be helped to do whatever is most right.

—TRADITIONAL AMERICAN INDIAN PRAYER

People who pray for miracles usually don't get miracles. But people who pray for courage, for strength to bear the unbearable, for the grace to remember what they have left instead of what they have lost, very often find their prayer answered. Their prayers help them to tap hidden reserves of faith which were not available to them before.

—RABBI HAROLD S. KUSHNER

LOVE—THE SACRED HEALER

This is my commandment, that you love one another as I have loved you.

—JOHN 15:12

According to Robert Wuthnow, "The quality of love in a group is the decisive element in fostering deep spirituality." When people see love and caring acted out in a group setting, they experience something sacred. People have difficulty putting the experience into words; they just know something very unique has happened to them as a result of the trust and the openness being modeled in the group. The warmth and the closeness of the group make people feel cared for and accepted. This experience leads people to sense that a higher power is more present and available in their lives. They reflexively connect deeds of kindness with faith and feeling closer to God.

Many of the world's most well known philosophers, psychologists, and theologians agree. Rollo May believed that love is the supreme value, united with will, which is the personal power to make love active in the world. Paul Tillich also stated that love is the supreme value, united with faith. He believed that love and faith give human beings the freedom and the courage to be themselves, to realize themselves, and then enable them to transcend themselves. Frankl also emphasized love. In *Man's Search for Meaning,* he wrote: "The truth is that love is the ultimate and the highest goal to which man can aspire. The salvation of man is through love and in love."

In the group environment, people experience a love that is given freely, a love that is not motivated by personal gain. When group members demonstrate love and caring among themselves, they contribute positively to one another's spiritual growth. In other words, they sense a divine presence among them, a sense that they have been a part of God's love.

Dossey believes that love and health are intimately related. If this is true, it would make sense that both human love and God's love make it possible for remarkable recoveries to take place, even when reasonable explanations fail to describe what has occurred. Regardless of the source of a person's pain, the love of others and the strength afforded by belief in a higher power can be a sacred source of healing.

Love is patient, love is kind.
It does not envy, it does not boast, it is not proud.
It is not rude, it is not self-seeking, it is not easily angered.
It keeps no record of wrongs.

Love does not delight in evil but rejoices with the
truth. It always protects, always trusts, always
hopes, always perseveres.
Love never fails.

—I Corinthians 13:4–8

Phase 3—In Search of Meaning

Though no one can go back and make a
brand new start,
Anyone can start from now and make a
brand new end.

From *As We Understood*, Alanon Family Group

By the time a group matures into Phase 3, most have created a
safe haven for one another and are ready to deepen their at-
tachments. Building on the solid trust level already established, sharing among the members becomes deeper and more
meaningful. People look forward to their meetings with expectation. They are genuinely interested in one another and
care about what happens to each member from week to week.
Each person is anxious to share his or her own news—whether
it is encouraging or discouraging. They want to hear how
others are getting along and are prepared to lend support to
whoever needs it. In return, they know they can also expect to
receive support and encouragement.

As people settle in, they learn to work together and to accept the various idiosyncrasies of each group member. Certain
group members become identified as leaders. Others remain
quiet and tend to be watchers. For the most part, however,
groups have generally progressed to a level of discussing sensitive issues and of helping one another find resolution of their
feelings. Honesty is a key factor during this period, and people

should be comfortable engaging in healthy conflict. When ground rules like nonjudgmental acceptance are emphasized, members are given permission to express their differences. The group's purpose is not to agree on all issues. People are encouraged to be themselves and to ask for what they want, without fear of being put down or ostracized. The overall purpose now is to provide a safe place where people can express their honest emotions without fear of judgment or retribution.

This phase of stability gives group members a chance to spend their time in a more focused and aligned way. People dig deeper for meaning and start to gain perspective on their life situation. Where at first they were paralyzed by the shock of crisis, now they may be able to assign some meaning to what has happened. By now, Dennis was clean and sober and was ready to assess the value of his experience. He was an active member of AA, past the stage of desperation, and committed to sobriety. He had fallen into a pattern of regular group attendance. Joan had recovered physically from the injuries sustained when she was struck by lightning. Once she and her husband were past the crisis point in their grief, they began searching for answers to difficult questions regarding the "why" of Jen's death. Joan needed spiritual healing to help her understand the tragedy better.

A word of caution is in order as the group moves into this phase. Don't get too comfortable! You run the risk of falling into a rut and stagnating. Some weeks, it may seem easier to just chat about current events or what ball team is winning or losing, or to exchange recipes. A little of this is acceptable because it's good to get a broad perspective on people's lives—where they live, what they read, how they think. But that's not the reason your group came together. Don't lose sight of your purpose. And if your purpose is learning to cope with a life crisis, remember that real growth still involves a little risk, pain, and uncertainty.

A stable group could be compared to a stable marriage. You're getting along fine, so why rock the boat? But novelty and change add spice to a marriage, and they can do the same for your group. For a married couple, a simple act like sitting in a different spot at the dinner table can remind you of how entrenched you are in everyday habits. Group members often sit in the same place as well. Think of creative ways to mix things up so your group stays excited about being together.

As a group, try to build on the strengths you have already developed, and remember that stagnation is a distinct possibility at this time.

STRUCTURE AND RITUAL

> This time, like all times, is a very good one,
> if we but know what to do with it.
>
> —RALPH WALDO EMERSON

Respect Your Rituals

The structure of your group is now pretty well established. You begin and end on time and repeat your ground rules as needed, especially when new people join the group. Your foundation has been solidified, and people know what to expect from week to week.

When you go around the circle and check in with each individual, you are participating in a ritual. By now, group members have an expectation of how the group is run. If you were to deviate, for instance, and bring in a speaker unexpectedly, you would throw off the normal routine and confuse your members.

After our Affirming Life group had been together for about six months, Donna and I had the opportunity to involve the group in Ingrid Dilley's Renewing Life pro-

gram. *The eight-week educational series is designed to enhance the quality of life of individuals who are chronically ill. We were excited about it and talked it up from week to week. I had made all the arrangements with the woman who would be teaching the class. We agreed we would do the class on Tuesday mornings, during our normal support group time.*

Imagine my surprise when the time came for people to confirm that they were planning to attend. Almost to a person, our group members chose not to go through the class. Was it the time commitment? Switching locations? Time of year? Donna and I never got a clear answer. But I believe part of the reason was that the class would have interrupted the normal ritual behavior of our group. Now that we had established a comfortable pattern from week to week, the group was reticent to change.

From this experience, Donna and I learned two valuable lessons. First, we should trust the wisdom of the group and be respectful of the rituals that have been created. Second, when we discussed what had taken place, we noted that the group had developed enough autonomy, trust, and honesty to rebel when the two facilitators tried to tell them what to do! They had confirmed (for themselves and for us) that this group belongs to the members, not the facilitators.

Closing Rituals

The Serenity Prayer

God grant me the serenity to accept the things
   I cannot change,
Courage to change the things I can,
and the wisdom to know the difference.

The inspirational reading at the end of our meetings has become an important part of our closure. This type of ritual provides a sense of belonging and closure to every meeting. In the first part of this chapter, you read about the sacred connections that occur in healthy groups. To reinforce this sacred connection, many groups utilize prayer, meditation, or relaxation as part of their ritual. Some close by reciting the Serenity Prayer. Others offer individual prayers at the end of the meeting.

Robert Wuthnow's surveys showed that prayer contributes significantly to the likelihood of people experiencing love and caring in a group. People tend to see love enacted through prayer. When they lift up a prayer for a member who is absent, they know that prayers will be coming their way on days when they cannot attend.

Spirituality as manifested in prayer is another way to find peace when facing difficult situations. Knowing you are not alone—that others care enough to pray for you—strengthens your faith that someone or something will take care of you in hard times.

Several other prayers and meditations are provided as part of the Discussion Guides at the conclusion of this chapter.

TECHNIQUES FOR DISCOVERING MEANING

In this phase of group development, group members can develop skills that help uncover the meaning behind each individual experience. Members can learn to search for the deeper meaning by asking probing questions or by interpreting the group's discussion. Through group sharing and interaction, each individual member learns a little more about himself or herself and how to assume responsibility for reactions and behaviors.

What is the purpose of probing? Through probing, we can actually enter the world of each group member, gather information, give information, and help that person take control of his or her situation. Probing is like peeling away the delicate layers of an artichoke one by one until you come to the soft and tender heart in the middle.

The Art of Asking Questions

> The shoe that fits one person pinches another; there is no recipe for living that suits all cases.
>
> —CARL JUNG

No two people in a group are going to think and act the same, even though they are in the group because of similar life situations. Skillful, probing questions help people to gain important information that helps them differentiate themselves from one another. Knowing when and how to use effective questioning can be a helpful tool in developing conversational skills. To put it more strongly, your group discussions are going to live and die based on the questions members ask one another or the facilitators ask the members.

Closed questions lead to one-word answers. They seldom allow a person to expand—Do you like to cook? (No.) Do you enjoy coming to the group? (Yes.) Have you been feeling okay? (Sometimes.) Closed questions rarely help group process, and facilitators should limit their use whenever possible.

Informational questions provide information about the person—What is your name? What loss have you experienced? When did it happen? These questions are necessary in order to get to know people, but they don't provide much insight into feelings.

Open-ended questions give the person an opportunity to talk about reasons, feelings, history, and so forth. This is the most effective questioning technique because it welcomes people's thoughts and feelings and does not limit their input— What was your first reaction to your cancer diagnosis? Why do you think AA helped you finally give up drinking? How have you managed to reconcile with God after the death of your daughter? These are difficult questions, but they do get to the heart of why people are in the group.

Feeling questions probe a little deeper than open-ended questions by asking about the individual's emotional reaction to an event—What do you feel now when a new member comes into AA? Now that two years have passed since Jen's death, how would you characterize your emotional health by comparison? When you learned that your cancer had recurred, what did that feel like inside? Obviously, feeling questions are the hardest to ask, but they do provide a window into that person's soul. When you answer a difficult question with an honest answer, you learn what is in your own heart and come to understand yourself better.

The Art of Interpreting and Responding

The group will benefit by understanding how to interpret what people say and by responding appropriately. What follows is a sample statement from a group member and a list of communication techniques that could be used to respond to this comment. By using these techniques, you can clarify and enlarge on your group's interaction and self-discovery.

Statement: "Last night, I told my best friend that my cancer has gotten worse and that I wanted to talk about my fear of dying. She said she didn't want to talk about it ... that I look just fine and that I worry too much. I felt bad."

Restating or rephrasing. When we listen to someone, we automatically interpret the person's words to suit our own thought process, taking into account the body language and the facial expression of the person speaking. When you respond by restating what you have heard, including the accompanying emotions, you allow the speaker an opportunity to either agree or disagree with your rephrasing. By doing this, you avoid miscommunication. A sample restating or rephrasing statement might be: "I hear you saying that you feel hurt when your friends won't acknowledge the seriousness of your illness."

Clarifying. To make sure you heard the person correctly, you might ask the person to explain further. A sample clarifying response would be: "I'm not sure I understand your concern. Did you feel bad because your friend doesn't really believe you are sick or because she didn't want to talk about dying?" When you ask for clarification, you let the speaker know you have been listening and that you understand that person's feelings but need to know more.

Interpreting. When you interpret, you offer possible explanations for certain behaviors, feelings, or thoughts. You are providing the speaker with a different perspective on what he or she has said, which encourages deeper self-exploration and perhaps a new understanding of his or her behavior. A sample interpreting response would be: "I'm thinking that perhaps your friend is feeling just as afraid as you are, that her way of dealing with her fear is to avoid it and not talk about it. What do you think?"

Giving feedback. When you give feedback, you express concrete and honest reactions based on your observation of *what* has been said and *how* it has been said. When you give feedback, you are uncoding the implicit messages the individual is sending, which helps that person make sense out of the experience. You also are helping the speaker to understand how the group as a whole might be viewing and/or understanding him or her. When giving feedback, be careful to get permission from the speaker: "Could I give some input on what I've heard?" Then focus on what you have observed, not your opinion of it. An example of feedback to the opening statement might be: "I sense that perhaps you are feeling abandoned by people who mean a lot to you when something like this happens. When we feel abandoned, we feel lonely. Do you sometimes feel alone with your feelings and your worries about dying?" Your feedback may increase the speaker's self-awareness and give the speaker a better understanding of how he or she appears to others.

Summarizing. If you want to close down a discussion or perhaps encourage further discussion with other group members, you can review the essence of what has been discussed. This shows the speaker that the group has been paying attention and gives that person a chance to respond with feedback. An example of summarizing the opening statement would be: "In general, we have probably all experienced insensitivity from family and friends at some time. Does anyone else have a comment?" This opens the discussion up to the group before closing the discussion.

Silence. When a conversation needs to be digested or is a cause for reflection, a constructive amount of silence can convey acceptance and support. Too much silence, however, can be uncomfortable and anxiety provoking. Use it wisely.

A Word to the Wise

Probing skills are wonderful tools—when used wisely. But they also can be overdone. We have probably all experienced situations in which the words "If I hear what you're saying . . ." have been used one too many times. The speaker begins to sound insincere—like an amateur psychologist—which can make people wary and reticent to continue sharing. Be sensitive, and try to tune into each group member's individual personality. Remember that most of communication is nonverbal. If a person's eye contact and body language tell you that he or she wants to explore further, continue to probe. Otherwise, leave well enough alone.

As Phase 3 progresses, the baton of leadership is being passed from the facilitator(s) to the group members themselves. In the beginning, the facililitators served as administrators and modeled group sharing skills. By now, group members should have learned to use those skills when interacting with one another.

CHALLENGES AND CONFLICTS

The Stagnant Group

By this phase, group members know one another well and have settled into a comfortable routine—perhaps *too* comfortable. Stagnation may occur for one or more of the following reasons.

1. Your group may have lost their sense of purpose. Why did they come together in the first place? Keep this focus alive and active at each meeting. At the start of each meeting, make sure that someone covers the ground rules and makes it a point to remind one another of the group's purpose and goals.
2. The group may be spending too much time on gathering and sharing *information* and not enough time on *feelings*. Make sure you are getting to the core of how each person feels about what is currently happening in his or her life.
3. One person's problem may be dominating each meeting, stealing from the group's cohesiveness and its goal of meeting every person's needs. If this happens, members should monitor themselves to make certain that everyone is having an opportunity to share. Allow time at the end of the meeting, if necessary, to refocus on one person's dominant need.
4. The group may become too large to accommodate meaningful dialogue. An ideal group size is 8 to 10 members plus two facilitators. Anything larger than this becomes cumbersome. Splitting the group up (family members and patients, husbands and wives, etc.) can be an effective solution to this problem. If this isn't feasible, you might consider dividing the group permanently and meeting at different times.

Helping Your Group to Grow

Group sharing should now be filled with more meaning and content. Help your group to grow and mature by making use of the following guidelines.

1. Give each person an opportunity to share. Don't allow one person to monopolize the group.
2. Avoid giving advice. People will discover their own coping mechanisms and techniques for regaining control of their lives and relating to others. Continue to use "I" statements.
3. Maintain a balanced discussion rather than getting stuck on one aspect of a subject over and over again.
4. Avoid blaming or finger pointing, in particular regarding specific physicians or the health care system. Try to stay positive and to focus on problem solving rather than complaining.

How do you know your group is coming together well? You will feel it in the way members communicate with one another. Sometimes, there will be more going on than you can keep track of. Generally, when you graduate from checking in around a circle to a give-and-take format in which everyone is contributing equally, you know you have made progress. The room will be filled with the emotions of life—laughing, crying, sharing, and caring. Through genuine caring for one another, the group finds meaning and hope. Now you have reached the group's spiritual core. Nurturing this spiritual core will deepen and strengthen the group's roots.

Discussion Guide #6
Defining Spiritual Needs and Spiritual Wellness

In a very basic way,
I feel God's presence with me
Like I have never felt before.
It creates a sense of calmness from within.

—ANONYMOUS

BACKGROUND MATERIAL

This topical discussion will focus on the power of a spiritual resource. Everyone has a different concept of God and of spirituality, but most people do believe in some form of inner power that helps them navigate rough seas. Be sensitive to the fact that some people may be offended by the introduction of religion into the group. The goal of this discussion is to help the group as a whole discover the strength that can come from recognizing a higher power.

To overcome any sensitivity, try to steer the discussion away from the narrow confines of organized religion, and attempt to find a broad definition of what the word *spiritual* means to each group member. Focus on the three aspects of spirituality presented in this section: connection, meaning, and hope. Spirituality also could be defined as a transcendent relationship between a person and that person's higher being. Or it may be defined as the inner resources of people, the ultimate concern around which all other values are focused, or the philosophy that guides their conduct.

In times of crisis, individuals may have difficulty establishing or maintaining a relationship with their higher being or higher power. They may feel abandoned by what they used to believe was a loving God. How do people know that their spiritual life is in trouble? When they feel empty, floating, devoid of purpose or meaning. People in true spiritual need no longer have a means for dealing with their own failures or shortcomings.

How can your group members confront these spiritual needs and work toward a spiritual wellness? By taking conscious steps to make sense out of their new lives. Spiritual wellness transcends the boundaries of organized religion and pursues a lifestyle that is life-sustaining and life-enriching. People who are alive spiritually *view* life and *live* life in a purposeful and pleasurable fashion. The following group exercise may help group members connect with the spiritual elements of their life.

GROUP EXERCISE

Distribute the handout at the end of this section, and use the following four elements as a way of initiating discussion of spiritual needs.

Ask the group to discuss their interpretation of the following topics and ways in which the topic is related to someone's spiritual life.

1. *Freedom of choice.*
   What are you free to choose in your life? What are you NOT free to choose? Are you currently taking advantage of the choices that you still have, regardless of the difficulty of your situation? How do you personally deal with the things over which you have no choice?

2. *Attributing meaning to life.*
   What meaning can you attribute to the life situation in which you find yourself? Has this been a wake-up call that allows you to reexamine life, to take a closer look at why you are here and the values you consider most important?
3. *Hope for the future.*
   What motivated you to become a part of this group? What did you hope for when you first joined? What do you hope for today? How has the group nurtured your hope? How are hope and spirituality interconnected?
4. *Connections.*
   Human beings long for connections. What connections did you have before joining this group? What new connections have you made? How are connections and spirituality interconnected?

SUMMARY

The goal of this discussion is to help the group identify their spiritual needs and find ways to strengthen each person's spiritual identity. Some people receive great strength from organized religion; others may have turned away from religion. This discussion is intended to help people see the larger elements of life that can provide meaning and pleasure for everyone, regardless of their religious affiliations.

Discussion Guide #7
The Meaning of Faith

Faith is the sense of life,
That sense by virtue of which man does not destroy
  himself,
But continues to live on.
It is the force whereby we live.

—LEO TOLSTOY

BACKGROUND MATERIAL

Children often ask probing questions: "Why?" "What's this for?" "What do I do with this?" As life progresses, either in times of trouble or in times of plenty, again we might ask the questions: "Why?" and "What do I do with this now?" Perhaps faith is the simple understanding that life is a mystery, and living in the mystery is what life is all about. Life is full of "what if's" and "why's." Faith helps us to accept life on its own terms and to believe that we can handle whatever comes our way.

Group members might use the following exercise to stimulate discussion regarding individual definitions of *faith* and ways in which faith has helped group members cope with their circumstances.

GROUP EXERCISE

Building on the preceding background material, ask group members to think for a few moments about the following statement:

> When you have come to the edge
> Of all the light you know
> And are about to step off into
> the dark of the unknown
> Faith
> Is knowing one of two things will happen:
> There will be something solid to stand on
> OR
> You will be taught to fly.

Ask people to define what the statement means in relationship to their life. Lead a discussion among group members regarding the differences among their definitions of the word *faith*. On a chalkboard or flip chart, summarize the responses. The goal of the exercise is to point out the individuality of spirituality and faith experiences. Regardless of how it manifests itself, however, some form of spirituality is inherent in human beings and tends to be the core from which faith emerges.

Faith is the realization that when we're alone . . . we are not alone.

SAMPLE MEDITATIONS AND PRAYERS

Lord, make me an instrument of Thy peace.
Where there is hatred, let me sow love.
Where there is injury, pardon.
Where there is doubt, faith.
Where there is despair, hope.
Where there is darkness, light.
Where there is sadness, joy.

O Divine Master, grant that I may not so much seek to be
    consoled as to console;
To be understood,
    as to understand,
To be loved,
    as to love;
For it is in giving that we receive.
It is in pardoning that we are pardoned.
It is in dying that we are born to Eternal Life.

   —ST. FRANCIS OF ASSISSI

Lord, what particulars we pray for,
    we know not, we dare not.
We humbly tender a blank into the hands of Almighty
    God;
Write therein, Lord,
What thou wilt, where thou wilt, by whom thou wilt.

   —THOMAS FULLER, *POEMS & TRANSLATIONS*

Lord God of mercies,
Grant to the souls of thy servants a place of cool repose,
The blessedness of quiet,
The brightness of light.
Through our Lord.

—ROMAN MISSAL

Faith consists in believing
When it is beyond the power of reason to believe.
It is not enough that a thing be possible
For it to be believed.

—VOLTAIRE

I do not seek to understand in order to believe.
But I believe in order to understand.

—ANSELM

Therefore encourage one another and build up each other,
    as indeed you are doing.

—THESSALONIANS 5:11

Chapter Five
Moving Forward—Giving Back

WISDOM FROM WOUNDED HEALERS

Have courage for the great sorrows of life and patience for the small ones. And when you have finished your daily tasks, go to sleep in peace. God is awake.

—VICTOR HUGO

What life means to us is determined not so much by what life brings us as by the attitude we bring to life; not so much by what happens to us as by our reaction to what happens.

—LEWIS DUNNING

On March 1, 1998, Kate attended a memorial service for Tim, a good friend and classmate who had died one year earlier in a tragic accident. He had been driving a sport utility vehicle when it went out of control and plunged over an embankment. The truck sank to the bottom of the Minnesota River, killing him and four other college students. His death had deeply affected her. "We grew up together, and he had always been a good friend," she remembers. "At our class reunion, he was worried about me. He suspected that my daughter's father was abusing me. He asked me when I was going to leave that jerk and marry him. I knew he truly cared and meant what he said."

After the memorial service, Kate went home—and the abuse began again. "I hid in the bathroom, locked the door, and prayed for strength," she says. Then, a feeling of calmness and courage came over her. She heard Tim's voice telling her to get out of there, that she deserved better. "I know he gave me strength to leave," Kate says. "I got up off the bathroom floor, packed my bags, grabbed my daughter, called the police, and left." Kate had been in denial about the abuse . . . until that day. "When I filed the order for protection, I had to list and describe the events leading up to that night," she remembers. "As I wrote them down, and then told them to the legal advocate, I was in complete shock. It took that experience to wake me up and see I was really being abused." Later that same day, Kate attended her first support group meeting.

"He abused me for the last time that night," she says proudly. In the past, she had always gone back to him. Now, with the support of her group, she has resisted that urge for more than one year. "One week was really hard—I felt like I had to go back so my daughter could wake up and go to bed each night with both parents. Then I went to my group, and they reminded me of all the reasons why I shouldn't go back." Kate was finally moving forward with her life.

GETTING RID OF FEAR

Kate took a huge step in her life when she filed the order for protection and walked out the door that last time. Yet she continues to live with fear and doubt. She knows that her progress forward must be measured one day at a time. "Each day, I wonder what lies ahead. Will I ever trust or fall in love with someone again? Will anyone accept me and my child?" She lives with almost constant anxiety. Some days, it's hard to get out of bed. At work, she escapes to the bathroom three or four times a day when she is overwhelmed with a need to cry. Flashbacks of the abuse continue to haunt her, and she lives in fear that it could happen again.

But today she is more confident than she was when she first started attending the group. That confidence gives her the strength to stay away from her abuser, even though she mourns the loss of her dream—a two-parent family for her daughter. "The group has helped me get to know who I am," Kate says. "During the four years of abuse, I had lost myself. I lived each day in fear."

Other women in Kate's group expressed similar feelings. Before coming to the group, many had come to believe that they could not make it on their own. Though they longed for freedom, the women had been alienated from other people and convinced by their abusers that it would be impossible to live without them. "Sharing with others gave me the strength and the boost to move on," is the way one woman summed it up.

Fear can be a constant companion for many people before they join a group. They felt very alone in their worries. Some believed they were the only ones suffering with this cancer diagnosis, the only woman who had ever been abused, the only parent who had suffered the loss of a child. Like Kate, they lived each day trying to avoid mistakes and to control anticipated difficulties. For many, their self-worth had plummeted.

Groups are extremely effective in helping people to address their fears and to learn to live with them. Sharing within the group can become an emotional safety net. A fear kept inside is multiplied. Giving voice to fear and listening to the group's counsel and encouragement helps to dissolve the fear's impact and makes it less powerful. Sister Arne summed it up when she said: "I have a fear which never seems to leave, especially after the recurrence. Just by saying it in support group, I felt hope and received encouragement because others have felt the same way and have learned to cope."

One of Dennis's most powerful lessons from AA is that he did not have to do it alone. Even though fears may be valid and normal, groups help people see that they do not have to solve them alone. Being able to trust and to feel safe in the group can translate into learning to be able to trust the world as well.

ONE DAY AT A TIME

Another member of Kate's group described her feelings after spending several months with the group. "Now I know I can do it—if I just keep trying—one step at a time." Their group helps the members see that they are not locked into a situation. "They help me see that, even though I'm living that way today, I don't have to live this way for the rest of my life."

Dennis and all other members of AA understand the constant threat of returning to a previous lifestyle of active alcoholism. The concept of living one day at a time is an integral part of their recovery. "Living in the future undermines my serenity," Dennis says. "When I live one day at a time, I accept God's help each day. Then I act accordingly and do what I know will continue to bring recovery and peace." And Dennis stresses that his experience is not unique. Millions of AA members are living successful lives—one day at a time.

The powerful motivator for most of them is the continued strength and determination they derive by attending group meetings. "In the group—the larger community—is where I *hear* God's will for me. God helps us through each other,"

Dennis says. "How I should live then becomes simple, mundane, and nonmysterious. Why? Because I see the members of my group living that sort of life—and being successful."

After a cancer diagnosis, the uncertainty of life becomes abundantly clear. For Donna, not a day goes by—even five years later—when she doesn't think about the potential of her cancer recurring. "Several years ago when I went on [the medication] Megace to prevent hot flashes, they warned me that I might gain weight," she says. "At the time I figured, what difference would it make? In my mind, I wasn't going to live anyway. Now, after five years, I'm starting to believe I'm going to live. And I'm still carrying around that thirty pounds." Donna is able to laugh at herself and the morbidity of her comment. It's difficult to not dwell on the what if's in life. But living one day at a time rather than in the past or in the future makes it easier to deal with the uncertainty.

LIVING IN THE MOMENT

Early in May, Sheri came to the group alone. Just one week earlier, during a follow-up visit to the Mayo Clinic, she and Randy had heard discouraging news. The tumors up and down Randy's spine were all larger. The doctors were even a little surprised to find that Randy hadn't experienced any numbness or tingling in his arms or legs. They warned him to expect symptoms in the near future. Sheri asked the doctors a series of difficult questions from a written list the group had helped her create: What will actually cause Randy to die? Is this the time to connect with hospice? Who should they call in case of an emergency? Both of them were mentally and physically exhausted by the time the day was over.

"We were devastated after hearing all the bad news," Sheri told the group. "So we escaped for the weekend." They found sitters for the children (one Grandma for the boys and another for Miranda) and headed to their parents' north woods cabin for the fishing opener. "Randy caught the biggest walleye of the weekend," Sheri said. "In a wheelchair, off the dock. It was a wonderful moment." While Sheri was visiting with the group that evening, Randy was trying his luck at angling one more time. A former co-worker had picked Randy up that morning, giving him the opportunity to spend a few more days up north.

In Randy's absence, Sheri was able to come to the group alone. It gave her a chance to catch her breath after an exhausting week. The predictability of the group's interaction—their laughter and joking—reminded Sheri of the stability that still existed in life, despite the chaos she had been feeling for the past week. The group also provided valuable information regarding how to contact hospice and encouraged Sheri to take care of herself by making those contacts as soon as possible.

Being a part of Sheri and Randy's life has helped each group member understand the importance of living in the moment. For many of us, our biggest mistake seems to be taking the ordinary events in our life for granted. In fact, those ordinary moments are the sacred essence of our being: The smell of a lilac bush in bloom or of cookies baking in the oven. Your child's bright smile getting off the bus on the last day of school. The feel of a walleye tugging on the end of your line.

Stopping to imagine Randy's joy as he pulls in one more fish, we might remind ourselves that *life is not a dress rehearsal.* Today is the only day you have for certain. Use it well. Savor time with those you love. Seek out the experiences that give meaning to your life.

> Even in the moment of looking back over one's life—even in the last moment—one is still there, experiencing, living. The present, not the future, is the eternal tense.
>
> —IRVIN YALOM

REACHING OUT—GIVING BACK

I don't know what your destiny will be, but one thing I do know: The only ones among you who will be really happy are those who have sought and found how to serve.

—ALBERT SCHWEITZER

Donna celebrated five years of cancer survivorship last year. As she blew out the candles on her cake, she paused to remember the myriad emotions she had experienced since first hearing the words, "You have cancer."

"At first, I felt a sense of unreality. I wasn't numb, just shocked. For several days, it was like living in a nightmare. I kept thinking, 'When will I wake up?' Then I cried every day for nine months. But I laughed every day as well! I was sad, afraid, terrified, overwhelmed, and exhausted."

Being a clinical psychologist, Donna doesn't believe she was ever clinically depressed. "I learned my spirit was indestructible—with a little help from family and friends." She also learned that a cancer diagnosis meant giving up on trying to control life. "Nothing in my life had ever come close to the profound powerlessness that having cancer produced."

Donna's original diagnosis was a rapidly multiplying breast cancer that already affected 15 of her lymph nodes. The statistics on five-year survival were not optimistic. After her mastectomy, Donna and husband Doug researched all treatment options and chose a peripheral stem cell transplant, which was considered experimental as a first-line treatment at the time. A major blood clot and infection during the treatment almost killed Donna. Six weeks of radiation followed. When it was all over, Donna tried to remain optimistic. But deep in her heart, she didn't believe she would ever blow out the candles on that five-year-survival cake.

Today, when my 12-year-old daughter asks me, "What does Donna do?" (as in, what does she do for a living), my reply is, "She lives." Donna *does* live each day. She balances her freedom to choose how she lives with her strong desire to help others faced with a similar challenge. She is a Reach to Recovery volunteer and coordinator. (Reach to Recovery is an American Cancer Society program that links breast cancer survivors one-on-one with newly diagnosed breast cancer patients.) She volunteers for HealthEast hospice. She has cofacilitated a breast cancer support group. And she came up with the idea for Affirming Life, the group for women with recurrent cancer, which has been meeting weekly for a year.

Now that her survivorship has stretched to five years, she sometimes asks the question "Why me?" in a positive, not a negative, context. Why is she the one to beat the odds and survive this long? Survivor's guilt (a common experience for many survivors) sets in as she watches group members die. Living her life in the shadow of uncertainty, Donna has discovered that reaching out to others provides meaning to her life. "In particular, I am very moved by the courage of the women in the Affirming Life group," she says. "And being a part of the group is my way of both giving back for all that I have received and preparing for what could be my future as well."

To learn to live without certainty and yet without being paralyzed by hesitation is to learn the lesson of acceptance.

—ANONYMOUS

CARRYING THE MESSAGE

In November of 1934, Bill Wilson was a washed-out Wall Street drunk. While in a detox hospital, Wilson experienced, by his own account, a sudden spiritual awakening. That awakening convinced him he could fully recover from alcoholism if he would be willing to believe in some power greater than himself. After a brief dry-out period, Wilson began pulling bowery drunks off bar stools and trying to convert them. After six months of failures, he said to his wife Lois, "Maybe I'm wrong about this spiritual thing being the answer." Her reply? "Oh no, Bill, you're absolutely right. You've never stayed sober this long." His belief in his program hadn't worked on the bowery drunks. But it had worked on Wilson.

He went on to pair up with Doctor Bob Smith, another supposedly hopeless drunk. On June 10, 1935, these two men founded what was to become the 12-step program of Alcoholics Anonymous and began carrying their message of hope to other alcoholics. Today, the program stretches across the world to 150 countries with 96,000 groups and several million members.

In some ways, carrying the message could also be characterized as reaching out and giving back. But Dennis views it as more than just that. "I don't carry the message out of obligation or altruism," he says. "Mainly, I do it because this is how I stay fresh and grateful. There is no way to truly understand the nature of spiritual recovery like trying to pass it on to someone else. The giving back is actually making yourself credible and attractive as someone who has been there and succeeded. It's something you do for yourself."

As Dennis tells it, every meeting is made up of a diverse cast of characters. On entering a room full of well-dressed, well-groomed people, a newcomer might wonder if he or she even belongs. "This person might be without a job, can't keep food down, thinks everyone hates him, and owes a million bucks," Dennis says. "Then, when I tell my story of being smelly, dirty, arrogant, and drunk some twenty-three years ago, that has an impact on this guy. I've made it for that long. Maybe he'll stay."

In AA, staying is a problem, according to Dennis, because the majority do not stay after their first meeting. "That's why you better be doing this for yourself," he says. "If you are filled with your own power—that you're going to keep this guy sober—you may be sorely disappointed. You do it because it's the right thing to do." As a result of this, new group members learn by example.

"The last thing drunks want to hear is advice," he contends. "They don't want you telling them what they should do. Rather, they want to see how *you* are doing." By welcoming newcomers, offering to be mentors and sponsors, and giving good example, AA members carry the message to others in an exemplary fashion.

For Dennis, the turning point in his recovery was the unswerving persistence of his three mentors. They taught him the true meaning of carrying the message through their example of dedicated sponsorship. "Although I refused to stay sober, they wouldn't leave me alone. They didn't bail me out of my drunkenness, but they also didn't show irritation with my arrogance or self-pity. They were never surprised that I was drunk, and admitted that the miraculous thing was their own sobriety. Thanks to that example, I have been sober for 23 years."

BECOMING CONFIDANTES

Mature groups cannot help but foster mature one-on-one relationships. Within the Affirming Life support group, two long-time friends attend the group together. Gwen is in her early seventies and is living with a recurrent lymphoma. Lea is in her sixties and continues to receive treatment for a breast cancer that has spread to her liver. They met as part of a church circle when they were both young mothers. Gwen laughs when she tells how the church group is still called the Young Mother's Circle, even though most members are now grandmothers. Through the years, the friendships that evolved from that group have transcended the group's initial reason for being—to meet the spiritual needs of young mothers. Today they meet to minister to each other's needs as older adults.

Gwen and Lea come to our group for a new reason—to discuss and to understand the feelings of women with recurrent cancer. But their history enriches this new wrinkle in both of their lives. They are already special friends. They know one another's families, respect one another's spiritual needs, and already know some of the intimate background leading up to this new cancer experience. Gwen and Lea help our group understand each of them better. In addition, they serve as a model for other group members. Through their long-standing friendship and genuine caring for one another, we see the possibilities in ourselves as potential confidantes.

I met Donna more than five years ago. I was cofacilitating the breast cancer support group that Donna joined shortly after her diagnosis. Almost from the beginning, we both sensed that we were destined to become confidantes. But her diagnosis was critical, and my role was to help facilitate her process. When she celebrated her third year of survivorship, my workload dictated that I resign my role as cofacilitator. I suggested that Donna take over. As a psychologist, she understood group process, and her own cancer experience would be invaluable as a facilitator. At that point, our relationship became more personal.

When her husband Doug was transferred to San Diego for two years, my husband and I visited them as part of our 25th anniversary celebration. When they returned to Minnesota, Donna and I worked together to establish the Affirming Life group. Our relationship as confidantes has been cancer's gift to both of us.

ACCEPTANCE—JUST AS I AM

Acceptance might be viewed as the net result of a healthy grieving process. For Joan, it will be the ability to finally recall her daughter Jen without intense pain. Dennis accepts that he is powerless to overcome his addiction without the help of a higher power. Donna accepts that cancer is a part of her life. People reach the point of acceptance by confronting their situations rather than denying them. Being a part of the group process allows this confrontation to occur. *Acceptance* doesn't mean liking the situation. It means you understand it better and are less fearful.

The pain of a life crisis will not vanish because you belong to a group. But the pain can be diminished and put in perspective. The group provides encouragement and resources to face what life brings. Each person in the group, especially those who have preceded you in a similar situation, can serve as a role model of what can be accomplished.

Jackie continues to serve as both a mentor and a model for Sheri. By her example, Jackie helps Sheri cope with each day's events, knowing that she is not the only one who has ever encountered this pain. Jackie provides physical support by babysitting and shopping, and she provides emotional support by sharing her own remembrances of Richard's time in hospice prior to his death.

"Next week, I've invited Sheri to come to my house and meet with the hospice nurse who took care of Richard," Jackie says. "Hearing what she has to say may help Randy and Sheri understand why signing up for hospice now would make sense for both of them."

As a result of being part of the Affirming Life group, Donna accepts and acknowledges the real possibility that her cancer could recur. Watching group members cope with recurrent cancer puts the situation in perspective. By observing their example, the reality of recurrence becomes less frightening. They are all living full lives—seeing grandchildren born, taking trips, directing choirs, working at full-time jobs, spending time in the garden, enjoying the moment. This observation helps Donna live each day in peace, knowing that she has confronted the reality of her fear without dwelling on it.

Acceptance means facing life with compassion and humility. We no longer struggle against life or try to control it. We no longer ask, "Why me?" To accept means to admit to vulnerability and mortality. Dennis and Donna understand what it feels like to be powerless. They know that being powerless does not diminish their humanity; in fact, it enhances that humanity. Despite painful circumstances, they have not been abandoned by life. Instead, their survival validates the goodness of life and the strengthening potential of a higher power.

MOVING FORWARD WITH FRESH PERSPECTIVE

Go confidently in the direction of your dreams.
Live the life you have imagined.

—HENRY DAVID THOREAU

Although many people remain in groups for years, others get their needs met and move on with a new perspective. Joan's experience serves as an example. "The next spring after Jen's death, our other children's ball schedules made it impossible to get to group meetings," she remembers. "When we returned in the fall, I was flooded with difficult memories. We had gotten so far in our grief journey, it was like starting over again." At this point, Joan wanted her grief to be more private. "I know that we would help other people by attending, showing that it does get better with time," she says. "But for me, it was just too hard."

Joan's spiritual journey meant moving on to a different kind of group. She would never stop grieving over her daughter's death, but she needed to attach some meaning to it and to discover how she could apply that meaning to her everyday life. Developing a Bible study group helped her accomplish that purpose. The knowledge she derives from the group and from her personal relationship with God helps Joan deal with the constant memory of what she has lost—and what she hopes to find again.

Dennis found himself falling away from regular AA attendance about six years after he became sober. For two years, he didn't attend meetings regularly. "I was working in a chronic pain clinic, which felt like a therapeutic treatment environment to me. I felt I was getting my needs met." He left the clinic and went into private practice in October. "By January, I was raving mad," he remembers. "I was eating and sleeping my job. I considered psychiatry—group therapy—looking at medical options. But in the back of my mind was this awareness; I knew what I should be doing."

Finally, he returned to AA. He was surprised to discover he was just as scared as at his first meeting. And this time, he wasn't drunk. "Here I was with seven years of sobriety, and I still felt crazy." The speaker that night shared a message that has stuck with Dennis ever since. "She talked about the second step—believing that a power greater than yourself can restore you to sanity," he said. "It was then I realized I needed a higher power just as much as before. When I was drinking, I drank and then went crazy. During the previous two years, I had been slowly going crazy. That had put me dangerously close to drinking again." After that pivotal meeting, the group became his home group and has been for the past 16 years.

LIFE LESSONS

What are the simple things that people have learned as a result of their group experience? "That family is so important," Jackie says, "so remember to say 'I love you' often." Jackie served an important role for Richard as he faced his death. In addition to keeping the house running, she was his major emotional support. "I needed the group for my own emotional support," she says. "They could buoy me up and make it possible for me to give all I had to Richard," she says. Her belief in the value of family and her altruistic desire to give back inspire her to help Randy and Sheri in any way she can. She does it selflessly, knowing the difference it makes in their lives.

For Sheri, the major healing factor the group provided was catharsis. Attending group meetings was an invaluable outlet for her emotions. "This is a place I can go—and need to go—to let out my fears, anger, and frustration. I can cry and be understood." Her most valuable gift from the group has been Grandma Jackie and the healthy perspective she sheds on Sheri's situation. "When I watch someone who has lost a loved one and see that she is making it—and helping me, too—I have hope that I can do the same some day."

Sister Arne's life lesson is the importance of finding a place of solace where you can share your deepest fears and concerns without being a burden to someone. "Even if I take the most time and talk in detail about my fears or my pain, the group always wants to help," she says. "If I feel guilty about something, they assure me that I'm doing what I can." The group also helped Sister Arne learn that humor is good medicine. For months, she had been telling the group how much better she was feeling as a result of eating artichokes. It became a weekly source of discussion. After her cancer recurred, the first thing Sister admitted to the group was that she was all done eating those artichokes. They hadn't worked as well as she thought. This bright spot in an otherwise somber discussion lightened the moment for everyone.

From her group, Kate has learned the value of loving yourself. "Women who have been abused don't feel lovable," she says. "We have been beaten down and told we are worthless. We have lost our identities. My group has helped me realize that you need to love yourself before you can give love to others." For the women in Kate's group, a reclamation of self was a valuable gift. Most had been isolated and convinced of their unworthiness. The group provided not only a safe haven, but also a mirror in which they could reflect on themselves. Once they reestablished a sense of identity, most realized that they were capable of independence without retribution from their abuser.

The lesson Joan learned from Compassionate Friends is probably the most valuable lesson of the support group experience—and the one that is repeated most often: *You are not alone.* "You can't imagine the sense of peace and comfort we took when we realized we were in a room with 10 other people who understood the incredible pain of losing a child," Joan says. This universality of experience heals like no other factor. It causes people to realize that there is no human deed or thought that is fully outside the experience of others. The common bond unites the group in community.

The most valuable outcome of the group experience for Dennis was his sobriety and the relationship he developed with his God and his community. After falling away from AA for a time, he also learned that his continued sanity was dependent on his association with his group. "I have learned that powerlessness is a constant state of being and one which we persistently deny," he says. "Recognizing and accepting that powerlessness over other people, places, and things was, and remains, a great relief for me. When I forget that lesson, my life returns to stress and misery."

Donna agrees with Dennis. "But despite the powerlessness I felt after having cancer, I also have learned from my group experience that the human spirit is unstoppable," she says. "People go on with courage in the face of incredibly difficult situations. When group members witness this kind of strength, it's contagious. We realize we have it within us to do the same."

A Community of Hope

"Hope" is the thing with feathers—
That perches in the soul—
And sings the tune without the words—
And never stops—at all.

—Emily Dickinson

Hope is never false. Although hope changes as circumstances and situations change, it still guards us against despair—no matter what. Support groups are communities of hope. You may enter the meeting room filled with despair and hopelessness. Rarely will you leave feeling the same way. The group's acceptance and lack of judgment will nourish you. They will take you in and love you just as you are. They will convince you that, despite the difficulty of your circumstances, you matter. You belong.

In the process, you just might discover a part of yourself that you never knew before—hope, that thing with feathers perched on your soul. The group's collective spirit has the power to capture you and convince you that hope is alive, just when you were feeling there was nothing more to do. No matter what you are hoping for, group members will listen and hope along with you. And because each group member is personally accountable to one another, most hopes expressed are realistic. When you are part of a group of individuals who are living a common experience, you will not easily move far from reality—the group will gently pull you back and remind you of it.

For Randy to hope for a cure would be hoping for a miracle. And that's okay. We should all expect miracles. But although the group supports his dabbling into unconventional medicine and his hope for a miracle (and prays for it to happen), they also encourage him to take advantage of the benefits of hospice and to be honest with himself about the reality of the Mayo doctors' prognosis.

Hope makes it possible to "let go and let God." By opening yourself up to a higher power, you learn to listen to your intuitive self and to trust that things might somehow work out. Hope is therapeutic and encourages you to try once more. Hope is your own personal cheering squad, your little engine that could. If you think you can, think you can, think you can—sometimes you just might be right. And even if you can't, the journey will probably be far more meaningful if you have a positive outlook regarding the possible outcome.

> Hoping is knowing that there is love; it is trust in
>   tomorrow;
> It is falling asleep and waking again when the sun
>   rises.
> In the midst of a gale at sea, it is to discover land.
> In the eyes of another, it is to see that she
>   understands you.
> As long as there is still hope, there will also be
>   prayer.
> And God will be holding you in his hands.

> —HENRY NOUWEN, *WITH OPEN HANDS*

LIVING LIVES OF PURPOSE

> He who has a *why* to live can bear almost any *how*.

> —FRIEDRICH NIETZSCHE

Mature groups are wise groups who understand that life is at times unfair and unjust. Most group members have lived through some form of adversity and understand the vale of tears. They stay together because they have discovered that the community spirit is a powerful source of strength. Their original reason for joining probably no longer motivates regular attendance. By now, most group members have confronted and dealt with the pressing need that brought them to group in the first place. Today, they are motivated by a desire to reconnect with people who matter—people they truly care about and want to help and support. Today, they are on a journey of self-discovery—to understand their own motivations and to make plans and goals for a hopeful future—and so they come to group meetings. The group helps them keep their journey on course.

Most members have discovered that in giving, they receive; that in loving, they truly experience love. One of life's true compensations is that it is almost impossible to help someone else without helping yourself at the same time. In a mature group, every person in the room has helped another person to navigate life just a little better. We would all be proud to have that as our epitaph.

In Handel's *Messiah,* one of the baritone solos tells the story of Christ being "despised, rejected, a man of sorrow and acquainted with grief." The people you have met in this book, each in a very individual way, can relate to this description. And because they have experienced life so completely, they are in a position to be of service to others. Through the process of group sharing, they have looked deep inside and fully exposed themselves to one another. They have shared their deepest darkness and their most painful wounds—as well as their brightest light and healing recovery. They have shared a spiritual journey of discovery. In the process, they helped one another separate the important from the unimportant, recognized the value of the moment, focused on love and the importance of relationships, and learned to accept their powerlessness and the strength of a higher power. They have reached out and lifted one another up. And in the process, they have been made whole.

As Rachel Naomi Remen concluded in her interview with Bill Moyers: "We are such a gift, each of us to each other, we human beings."

Whatever comes, this too shall pass away.

—ELLA WHEELER WILCOX

PHASE 4—IN SEARCH OF THE FUTURE

Like human beings, groups mature and gain wisdom with age. In the infancy stage, groups are groping to understand their purpose, and facilitators act as parents: They establish a structure for the group and provide a safe environment so group members can learn to trust. As the group evolves into adolescence, members begin grasping for their place, asserting their independence, and learning to understand one another's idiosyncrasies, including their strengths and weaknesses. Although they have come together for a common purpose, they soon learn that their personal beliefs and coping mechanisms may be quite different. During this stage, the facilitators act as coach and referee, acknowledging the differences among group members and encouraging honest dialogue.

By the next stage, the group is growing in maturity. A core group usually has developed, and individuals have reached a comfort level with one another. Often, group members have assumed certain roles. One person might be the peacemaker, whereas another is the critic. One person might bring articles filled with information, and another enjoys reading poetry or inspirational stories. Certain people initiate most of the dialogue; others are more comfortable responding. In this stage, facilitators act as instigators, shaking things up a little. They change the format of the meeting once in a while, or they take the group on a field trip. At this point, groups try to avoid stagnating and getting into a rut.

When a group has fully matured, a sense of synergy emerges. The group is now truly a circle of friends. Group members have come to understand that membership in this circle is a two-way street. Individuals benefit from group support, but each individual's contribution is a direct benefit to the group as a whole. As each person becomes healthier, the group as a whole benefits and becomes healthier. Most members now look forward to group meetings with great anticipation. You can feel the energy as you enter the meeting room. People greet one another warmly. They get updates on long-standing personal situations. Most come prepared to discuss specific issues.

In the mature group, the rigid roles that people may have assumed begin to fall away. The skeptic makes an effort to be a peacemaker. The grumpy complainer could surprise everyone by telling an emotional personal story that moves them to tears. Even 12-step groups, which typically have a strict format, might deviate from their normal order to just spend time talking freely with one another.

SUSTAINING THE MOMENTUM

This is a time for group leaders to sit back and feel proud of what has evolved. Their desire and willingness to cultivate the group are now paying off. To sustain this synergy, leaders and group members might think about using the following tools to sustain the group's momentum.

Remember to share and to give positive feedback. In the mature group, sharing takes on a new meaning. Sharing can mean sharing of responsibilities, of leadership, and of your time. The more that individual group members share in the care and maintenance of the group, the more they can claim ownership in the group. And when a member does something above and beyond, remember to give positive feedback. Human beings thrive on praise, a natural boost to self-esteem. When someone offers especially meaningful encouragement and understanding to another individual, be sure to provide praise. This is a very effective way to let the group know that their work is being accomplished. Hearing another person praised encourages the group to contribute. Remember, however, that empty praise is worse than no praise at all. Use the technique sparingly and only when the situation warrants.

Identify common themes and experiences as they emerge. One of the most important healing qualities of support groups is having each person learn that he or she is not alone, that other people are thinking the same thoughts and feeling the same feelings. In the mature group, the common themes become more intimate and complex. For example, in the early phases of our Affirming Life group, death was rarely discussed. As the group evolved, and we watched one of our members become more ill and finally be put under hospice care, we became more comfortable discussing this difficult, but very common, theme: our thoughts and fears about death. Bringing this topic to the forefront for discussion removes its stigma and allows group members to get rid of the loneliness and isolation of their private thoughts about a subject that is on all of their minds.

Hold one another accountable. Groups gain their strength and energy in a circular rather than a linear pattern. The resulting synergy is highly unlikely in one-on-one interaction. Think about the group of individuals you consider your friends. Do they know one another? Are you the same person with each of them? If you and your closest friends were all in the same room together, how would you act? Most of us have friends—but in many cases, our friends don't know one another. That means we don't necessarily have to be accountable. We can act one way with a childhood friend but perhaps in a totally different way with a newly found friend.

Mature group members are accountable to one another. Accountability forces people to think about their actions and the consequences of their behavior. One of the positive outcomes of this accountability is that a person's core self begins to emerge. By using the group as a sounding board and a mirror, members begin to see and to understand themselves better. When they express innermost thoughts and feelings out loud, in a safe environment, they clarify exactly what is important to them—and what is not. When members listen to themselves and see the group's reactions, certain patterns emerge.

Connect similar group members. Thanks to the magic of intuition or chemistry, some group members will naturally gravitate toward one another. Two people may have more in common with one another than with the rest of the group, and such pairs probably have the potential to become confidantes in addition to being fellow group members. These special one-on-one relationships can be an important part of the group's spiritual development, because connections are a key part of spirituality.

In today's society, where people are so busy working, connected only by computers most of the time, many are longing for new, meaningful friendships. Yet they are uncertain where or how to find them. Involvement in small groups is an excuse for that friendship to develop. And because people joined the group for a specific reason, some pairs already have distinct similarities. If you sense that two people might become confidantes, invite conversation between them. Help them explore the potential connection between them.

Summarize the group experience. As it evolves, the group may occasionally wonder if it is making progress and continuing to serve its mission. Summarizing group learnings and the themes that have emerged over the months validates the group members' importance to one another. A meeting specifically designed to talk about the group's direction may be particularly effective when the wind seems to have gone out of the group's sails and they have lost direction. At this point, the facilitator might develop a meeting agenda that asks each individual to discuss how his or her life has been enhanced by group membership. The group can leave that meeting with these individual accomplishments foremost in their memory.

Share leadership responsibilities. By now, the facilitator's role has shifted from leader to cheerleader. For some facilitators, it can be hard to step away from the leadership role and to let the group manage its own interaction. But the most effective groups are ones that have become self-governing. Now is the time for the facilitator to stay out of the way and let the group manage itself—to relinquish control and become part of the whole—and then watch as new leadership emerges.

Summary. Enjoy the learnings that derive from each group meeting. Help to cultivate one-on-one friendships and the growing relationships between confidantes. Encourage people to call or correspond with members who have fallen away. Continue to facilitate group process, when necessary. Take responsibility for introducing new members and helping them to feel comfortable. Be on the lookout for disruptive conflict or stagnation. In general, just enjoy.

But always be prepared. Groups are not stagnant. Your group's final destination is still uncertain. Although the group may continue indefinitely using the current format, group members might want to expand and develop programs that serve the larger community. Most people have a desire to give back to the community in some way. Your group may still expand its purpose, segment into smaller groups, or disband entirely.

SERVING THE LARGER COMMUNITY

According to the helper-therapy principle, giving help to someone else is the best way of being helped. This occurs because the helper feels good that he or she has something to give. By giving to someone else, he or she automatically becomes less dependent and more in control. When the group does something useful for society, they are collectively empowered. This type of behavior can emerge naturally from a mature group in which all the individuals are comfortable with their own personal development. Timing is critical, however, because it is difficult for people to reach out and give back before they are effectively healed themselves.

Alexis de Tocqueville believed that small groups might be the key to helping a society deal with its larger social issues. "Race for the Cure," an outgrowth of the work of the Susan B. Kommen Foundation, is a hugely successful event that grew out of one woman's desire to make a difference. Nancy Brinker watched her twin sister, Susan B. Kommen, die of breast cancer. Later, when Brinker was diagnosed with breast cancer herself, she set out to establish a program to fund research toward a cure. Today, many of the women and families who participate in the annual event have mobilized out of small support networks across the nation. But their collective impact and visibility have greatly affected the public's perception of this problem. And funding for breast cancer research has increased, from both the private sector and government programs.

Individuals who did not have access to groups also make similar contributions by turning their suffering into a mission that serves society. Gavin de Becker, a contributing editor for *USA Weekend*, grew up in a violent world. His mother's heroin addiction resulted in violence and abuse for him and his siblings. "It was my job to be sure the family got through those years alive," he remembers. His mother committed suicide when he was 16. But years later, de Becker realized why he had invested so much energy in the prediction and prevention of violence—to help others. Today, he is a personal safety expert. His two books, *The Gift of Fear* and *Protecting the Gift* were written to help others understand and trust their own intuitive protection mechanisms, for themselves and for their children.

In most groups, a majority of the members work within the group to help other members in need. The millions of people whose lives have been saved by AA are called to help one another. By overcoming debilitating addictions, people are healthier and more capable of living productive lives in the larger world. Groups help their members to gain perspective and control of their problems. When people are freed from self-doubt and insecurities—whether they are the result of a death, illness, addiction, or abuse—they are then empowered to reach out to others.

WHY GROUPS TERMINATE

Many open-ended groups sustain themselves for years. People move in and out, based on their needs; but a core group always seems to remain at the heart. If the original facilitators stay with the group, they help it evolve through different generations of members.

Sometimes, however, even the most intimate, close-knit groups reach a natural ending point. If the group makes it through all four phases of development, the whole group will sense intuitively that their mission has been accomplished. This holds true more for grief groups than for groups for people with chronic illness or chemical dependency.

When group members sense that the group is falling apart, they should talk about it honestly. Initiate a frank and open discussion of what is happening, how the group might be saved, or whether the group is ready to disband. The positive aspect of disbanding is that perhaps each person is ready to move on to a new level in their spiritual journey.

HINTS FOR CLOSING THE GROUP

By phase 4, the relationship among facilitators and group members is usually quite strong. A satisfactory closing will help everyone maintain their gains and continue to grow. A less than satisfactory ending could feel like a door slammed shut; a good ending could feel like a new beginning.

Powerful commitments require clear acknowledgment of their ending. For this reason, the final meeting should be well planned: It might take the form of a ritual to commemorate the group's value and success, or members might be asked to speak about what the group has meant to them and why each person believes it is terminating. Think about making the following elements a part of that closing.

Close any unfinished business. During your group's tenure, you have undoubtedly covered a wide variety of issues. Some of them may be unresolved. This last meeting is a time to wrap things up—to discuss those lingering topics and to see if resolution is possible. For instance, a group member may be searching for a new vocation or experimenting in a new relationship. Acknowledge these things and provide encouragement. A simple statement might be: "We know you're looking at a new job (or you are spending a lot of time with a new friend). Maybe you'll let one of us know how things work out." This closes that unfinished business, even though the situation is ongoing. Closure lets each person know their well-being is in the thoughts of other group members, even if the group is no longer meeting.

Add up the learnings and reflect on the experience. What has this group learned from one another? What are the common themes? Where is each member now compared to when the group started? To what do members attribute their growth? What roadblocks, if any, have they encountered? What are their goals for the future? Personal reflection on the part of each group member will create a meaningful group closure and will help each person understand where he or she is on their own spiritual journey.

For this last meeting, the facilitator once again assumes a leadership position because this reflection might be more effective if it is somewhat structured. This is a time for the group to be introspective, to identify specific ways the group has helped them to grow.

Help transfer skills to life. The strengths that have been built up as a part of this group experience will translate into each person's ability to deal more successfully with life in general. Discuss the gains made—whether in self-esteem, communication skills, personal insight, or community altruism. Identify specific coping skills that members can now build into their lives.

Identify ongoing support systems and resources available. For those who wish to continue a group experience, identify what is available in the community and ways to access the proper resources. The Internet information in the next chapter may prove helpful.

Connect people with one another in an informal way. Prepare a list of the names, addresses, and telephone numbers of all group members, and distribute them at this meeting. Suggest community events that may be of interest to all group members, and encourage people to go together. Identify other appropriate educational opportunities.

Some of the people you have met in this book remain committed to their groups. Others have fallen away. But the benefits they derived from the experience will be long-lasting. Endings can also be viewed as beginnings. Wisdom comes from wounded healers. In the first half of this section, you learned the insights of several group members as they personally examined their endings and beginnings. As you reflect on their lives, I hope you recognized parts of your own life and learnings as well. Shalom.

Discussion Guide #8
Defining Crisis and Understanding the Grieving Process

Keep a green tree in your heart
And the singing bird will come.

—CONFUCIUS

BACKGROUND MATERIAL

The Chinese language uses two characters to define the English word *crisis*—one of the characters means "danger" and the other means "opportunity." The Chinese understood that, beyond the initial danger presented by a crisis, opportunities were possible. Similarly, support group members encourage one another to look beyond the danger of their situation and to begin searching for the opportunities that can result from the crisis.

Getting past the danger of crisis requires time and effort. The first step might be adding up the losses and taking a close look at the impact. This examination may closely parallel the stages of grieving that occur after losing a loved one: (1) shock, (2) denial, (3) reaction, (4) mobilization, (5) acceptance.

GROUP EXERCISE

Use the five stages of grief to initiate discussion. Write down each stage on a flip chart or chalkboard, and ask for personal reactions and examples from group members who have either experienced that stage or who feel they are in that stage now. Record group members' answers. Consider summarizing the findings of the discussion on a handout and passing it out at the next meeting. The following questions might stimulate discussion about each stage.

1. How did you know you were in shock? What were the physical symptoms? What were you feeling emotionally?
2. How did you or a family member recognize that you were in denial? What did you do to get back in touch with reality?
3. *Reaction* means that reality finally sinks in and a variety of emotions begin to surface—anger, fear, depression, and so on. What did you feel first?
4. *Mobilization* means action. What action did you take (or do you intend to take) to move forward into the future?
5. For those who have reached the acceptance stage in their grieving process, what coping strategies have you developed to get to this stage?

Help group members understand the importance of enacting a plan that involves the following steps: (1) accept the reality of their loss; (2) experience the pain of their loss; (3) adjust to a new and changed environment as a result of the loss; (4) reevaluate and restructure, then move on into a new and changed life.

SUMMARY

Getting beyond the danger of a crisis to the point where opportunities become apparent is made easier by understanding the natural grieving process. The goal of this discussion was to help group members to identify where they are in that process and to give them an opportunity to share their coping strategies with one another.

Discussion Guide #9
Identifying Opportunities Arising from Crisis

BACKGROUND MATERIAL

In the normal course of life, people can easily fall into complacency and take life for granted. In the wake of a life-changing situation, however, people are forced to re-assess their lives. German philosopher, poet, and critic Friedrich Nietzsche said, "He who has a why to live can bear almost any how." Victor Frankl, a Holocaust survivor, discovered that those who find meaning in their lives are the strongest survivors. Meaningful activity that capitalizes on people's interests and gifts can provide the impetus to keep going during difficult transitional times.

Coping is a part of the normal grieving process. Group members can help one another to accept and to learn how to live with their changed lives. Some might choose to be angry and miserable. Others might choose to see new opportunities for growth as a result of the life-changing event. A key difference between these two reactions is the ability to find purpose in life and to assign meaning to your activities.

GROUP EXERCISE

Building on the background material, prepare the following list of questions and hand them out to group members. Ask the questions verbally as well as listing them on a flip chart or chalkboard. The goal is to help people identify their life purpose through answering the questions.

1. What kinds of activities do you find stimulating, satisfying, enjoyable, or just plain fun?
2. Try to remember a time when it felt like you were in the right place at the right time. What were you doing?
3. What do you naturally do well?
4. What do you daydream about doing?
5. Do you have a cause or an issue about which you feel passionately?
6. What would you attempt if you were certain you would not fail?

The goal of this exercise is to get people thinking about their unique talents, interests, and gifts. Encourage group members to take the questions home, to consider them carefully, and to look for their life's purpose through the answers. Sometimes a willingness to change is a key factor in achieving this life purpose.

SUMMARY

Opportunities can arise as a result of crisis. This discussion guide is designed to help group members to identify what gives meaning to their life—their true life's purpose.

Discussion Guide #10
Reaching Out to Relationships

It takes a great soul to be a friend.
One must forgive much, forget much, forbear much.
It costs time, affection, strength, patience, love.

—A. PURNELL BAILEY

BACKGROUND MATERIAL

After a life-changing event, people naturally expect to receive support and understanding from those closest to them—spouse, children, or friends. But remember that those individuals are riding the same roller coaster and experiencing the same feelings. If you are shocked, so are they. The same goes for anger, fear, denial, and guilt. And when two people are both angry or afraid or feeling helpless, their ability to communicate is handicapped. To regain control of these feelings, people must learn to share them with the the most important individuals in their lives.

A large part of going forward with life involves re-establishing important relationships—and perhaps building new ones based on common experiences. Yet, it is understandable that for many people, reaching out can be frightening. Fear of rejection may stop them from making the first overture.

Remind your group that healthy relationships will facilitate the healing process. Encourage them to take the risk.

GROUP EXERCISE

Building on the background material, ask group members to prepare a "gratitude list" of people who have made a difference to them. The list should include specific things the people on the list have done to help the group member deal with their current life situation. Give the group adequate time to prepare the list. Then ask if anyone would be willing to share their list with the group. After listing a few items on a flip chart or chalkboard, point out how these lists clarify the importance of human connections.

Encourage group members to share these lists with the individuals to whom they are grateful. Remind them of how this type of interdependence can help the healing process. Suggest that they also reach out to a special relationship before the next meeting—perhaps someone who belongs on their gratitude list, but with whom they have not spoken for some time. Plan on doing group sharing around this activity next time.

Chapter Six
Surfing the Net for Support
The Pros and Cons

The Internet can be a valuable resource for people seeking support. By surfing the Net, you can find educational materials and social contact with others in a similar situation. This section provides background information on the Internet and practical suggestions for accessing the support you need.

WHAT IS THE INTERNET?

The Internet is an international network of computers. The World Wide Web ("WWW" or "the web") is a system that provides information through the Internet, making it easier for individuals to access the Internet.

- *Chat groups* or *discussion groups* or *online support groups* provide forums through which people can communicate with other people and can share experiences and coping strategies.
- *Home pages* are web sites created by individuals, agencies, or organizations that can contain practically anything. Some describe personal experiences through stories, poetry, or artwork. Others include referral information about resources for support, such as peer support groups and

counseling services. Many sites contain an electronic-mail (e-mail) address through which you can correspond with the individual, the agency, or the organization.

How Can I Access the World Wide Web?

You need two things to connect to the World Wide Web: (1) a computer with a modem (either internal or external) and (2) an online provider for connecting to the Internet. Some national commercial providers (like America Online—AOL) sometimes offer free trial subscriptions. Some providers service local geographic regions. To find an Internet service provider (ISP), look in your Yellow Pages or in the classified ads in your local newspaper under "computer services" or "Internet providers." Sometimes, community-based organizations known as "Freenets" provide free services. Look in the computer section of your local library or bookstore for useful hints for choosing an Internet provider. Be sure to choose a provider with a *local telephone number* (or "dialup") to avoid long distance phone charges.

If you do not own a computer, you may get access through a local public or university library. A community health resource center, a medical school library, or a friend with a home computer may also be able to help you. If you are not able to gain free access, some copy centers and "cyber cafes" (coffee shops that rent computers by the hour) sell Internet access time.

What Should I Do When Looking for an Online Support Group?

Be patient and take your time. Sometimes, due to unusually high traffic, Internet access may be completely unavailable, or information may be slow coming. If you are not comfortable with computers, try to search with someone who is used to them. Look over the variety of "browsers" or "search engines" available to you. Usually, you can search one of two ways. (1) If you know an exact address (www.cancercare.com), you can type it in and go directly to that site. (2) If you are just looking for a general category, you can type that category into a search engine and ask it to look for possible sites. Define your key words as specifically as possible. For example, if you are interested in starting a support group for people with depression, you would probably yield too many files by typing in "depression." On the other hand, "depression and support groups" may give you a more narrow selection.

You could spend hours—even days—wading through all the information. Some sites offer automatic links to related sites. Be selective; if you do not have free access, costs can accumulate quickly. And be cautious; anyone can post information on the web. Be a wise consumer. Make sure that the information comes from an accurate and reliable source.

Every month, many new sites are added to the Internet that provide information, resources, and online support. In particular, sites like the Self-Help Clearinghouse and the National Organization for Rare Disorders, Inc., provide very reputable information about support groups, different diseases, newsgroups, and related web sites.

If you are unable to attend a local support group, cannot find one, or are uncomfortable being with people you don't know, you can receive reassurance and encouragement from an online support group. Options vary from small, chatty groups started by "just folks" to other sites that are jam-packed with information about your life situation.

- **The American Self-Help Clearinghouse (www.cmhc.com/ selfhelp/)** is a comprehensive, reliable site that will guide you to over 700 support groups, plus information about starting new ones. This site has just about everything, including first-person stories and an endless supply of great professional articles.

- In the Self-Help Resource Room, you will find a lengthy list of diseases and health problems with their related web sites. Clicking on any of these individual sites connects you with other resources, including organizations that are dedicated to your cause.

- **The National Organization for Rare Disorders, Inc. (NORD) (www.nord-rdb.com/-orphan)** maintains a data base of 5,000 rare disorders and disabilities. Searching the database gives you a description of the disorder and links to information about related disorders, organizations, and support groups.

- **The Health Show (www.tv.cbc.ca/healthshow/support/ listing.html)** offers a list of online support groups under general topic headings. Also listed, when available, are the frequently asked questions (FAQs) compiled from the groups. They recommend reading through the FAQ list before taking the time to join the group.

- A Canadian Internet site through **Sympatico: Healthy Way Magazine (www.bc.sympatico.ca/Contents/Health/ HEALTHYWAY/feature_sel2.html)** contains several interesting articles about self-help groups, plus other excellent HealthyWay Health Links. Some of their other sites include *About Self-Help and Self-Help Resources, Friends' Health Connection, On the Road to Healing, Psychology Self-Help Resources on the Internet, Starting an On-Line Self-Help Group,* and many others.

- For links to sobriety and recovery, the Sobriety and Recovery Resources page **(www.winternet.com/~terrym/sobriety. html)** has an extensive listing, including several AA-related web links, online meetings, chat channels, and mailing lists.

Musa Meyer's book *Holding Tight, Letting Go: Living with Metastatic Breast Cancer* evolved from a very well-developed online support group for women dealing with recurrent disease.

Through their ongoing dialogue, these women became like family. After several years, several of the women and their spouses made arrangements to meet, and they spent a wonderful weekend getting to know one another in person.

Sometimes the endings are not so bright. One man allegedly confessed to killing his daughter in an online mailing list. He was a member of an online alcoholism support group. Some group members felt his confidentiality had been compromised when he was indicted as a result of the listing. The man who notified authorities was saddened by such a reaction. He couldn't believe that more people couldn't see that the fact he had committed murder was more significant than his confidentiality.

Ethical and legal issues aside, there is still the growing debate over whether online support groups are actually helping people overcome their problems or not. Most chat rooms, newsgroups, and online forums have little or no professional guidance, and the people who run them may have little or no training in counseling or therapy.

Sometimes, the anonymity of the Internet works against finding real people and real support. People can create an Internet personality and hide behind it rather than confront their own personality defects and try to overcome them. This is one reason why Narcotics Anonymous does not sanction online meetings. They believe that nothing parallels sitting down and looking someone in the eye. Credibility seems to be the major problem on the Internet. Let the buyer beware.

Security can also be an issue. People must be cautious about giving out names, addresses, telephone numbers, and other information that could be dangerous if placed in the wrong hands.

Because I have spent so much time in one-on-one support groups, I have a strong bias about the power of face-to-face human contact. Nothing can compare to the touch of a human hand or the healing quality of a human smile. In a world where everyone and everything is wired, I hope we can continue to find ways to connect and to support one another—in person.

Chapter Seven
P.S. So You Want to Be a Group Leader

GETTING ORGANIZED

This book describes the powerful connections that take place in successful small groups and clearly explains the importance of the connections among kindred souls. But successful groups don't just happen. Committed leaders take the initial steps to get these groups organized and foster their growth. This section of the book is a step-by-step program to help you successfully develop a program that turns strangers into a community of friends.

First impressions are often lasting impressions, which is why it's important to get a group off to a good start at the very first meeting. When everyone is new, group leaders/facilitators must work hard at helping all group participants feel welcome and comfortable. *Give your first meeting careful thought—and come prepared.*

This section provides tips on group structure, format, and rituals. Anecdotes on real group happenings are provided to clarify each point. A facilitator's leadership skills, attitude, and genuine warmth are all extremely important to a group's success—starting at the very first meeting.

Tip One
Get Organized and Be Properly Prepared

Ten minutes before the first group meeting begins, a good facilitator should have nothing left to do. That leaves him or her free to greet any early arrivals or to spend a few minutes reviewing the format for this first meeting and the initiation of the discussion. When group members arrive, they deserve the facilitator's undivided attention.

> We learned this lesson in spades at our initial Affirming Life group meeting. We were due to start at 11:30 A.M., so Donna (my cofacilitator) and I agreed to meet in the cafeteria at the hospital at 10:45 A.M. That would give us time for coffee and for comparing notes on how the meeting would be run. By 11:00 A.M., our first group member had arrived! We were thankful that the room was open and that we were ready, free to spend that extra time getting to know our first group member.

Tip Two
Create a Warm and Welcoming Environment

The ideal is for your group to meet at the same place and in the same room every time. Make sure the location is well posted. Arriving at a building and not knowing where to go to can make people feel unwelcome. Post signs liberally, and (if applicable) let the people at the Information Desk know what is happening and where you will be.

Design the room for the anticipated size of the group—a group of 6 would probably feel swallowed up in a room set for 20, and a group of 20 would be very uncomfortable in a room for 6. Because circles imply connections, try to seat individuals in a circle—whether around a table or just sitting in chairs or on couches. People should be able to make eye contact with everyone else in the room.

Posters are an inexpensive way to brighten a room, and you probably have some favorite posters that would be appreciated by your group. At the outset, make certain people either have name tags (if sitting informally at chairs) or name "tents" to place in front of them on a table. This makes it possible for each person to personalize his or her comments to other group members without grappling to remember their names. Try to avoid a room with glaring fluorescent lighting. If you're stuck with fluorescents, at least turn off a few lights to soften the environment. You'd be amazed how just a touch of atmosphere creates a comfort zone for anxious group members.

After our first Affirming Life group meeting, I sent out a brief evaluation form to the women who had attended. One comment came back asking if we could have coffee at every meeting. For many people, coffee and "something for the other hand" (cookies, bars, etc.) is a comforting part of a group meeting. At the church where I grew up, social discussion took place in "fellowship hall" and always involved refreshments of some sort. Breaking bread (or a lemon bar!) together is a part of true fellowship.

In December, our Affirming Life group used one meeting to celebrate the season. I brought a tablecloth, candles, hot homemade soup, and a cassette tape player so we could enjoy seasonal music. To this day, we remember that meeting as one of the high points of our group development.

Tip Three
Meet People at the Door with a Personal Greeting

Strong eye contact, a friendly hello, and a handshake are the beginnings of a trusting and caring relationship between a facilitator and his or her group. Again, emphasize that people wear name tags, and work hard at memorizing faces and names right away because personalizing the welcome can help develop an early bond. The facilitator who comes to the second meeting knowing each person's name (before they put on a name tag) confirms his or her interest and strengthens that bond.

> *In my early thirties, with a new baby and another on the way, I felt a need to reconnect in a church setting. I attended St. Andrew's Lutheran Church several times. One Sunday, I was not wearing a name tag. As I was making the obligatory march down the aisle at the close of the service to shake hands with the pastor, I was amazed to hear him say, "Hello, Linda." I was sold.*
>
> *Much later, during a casual conversation with Pastor Eigenfeld, he shared his philosophy. "I know that if I can personalize my greeting to someone at the close of the service by remembering that person's name, it is very likely I have a new member." He was right. His congregation is now one of the large "megachurches" in Minnesota.*

Tip Four
Establish Group Norms

Starting and Ending on Time Facilitators can establish a safe, protective environment for new group members by adhering to a certain set of group norms, beginning with a predictable start time and end time for every group meeting. If the advertised start time is 7:00 P.M., then the meeting should start right at 7:00, even at the risk of having people arrive after the meeting has started. This establishes a clear expectation for everyone. Activities should be planned carefully so you can also close at the announced time.

Facilitator Introductions Facilitators can begin by introducing themselves and by stating their personal connection to the group's purpose and their reason for becoming a facilitator. Personalizing this introduction helps create a comfort zone for members. Try to make eye contact with every group member during this introduction.

Housekeeping Details At the first meeting and at subsequent meetings when new people have joined, cover general housekeeping items, which may include the following:

- Details regarding parking and handicap access information.
- Location(s) of rest rooms.
- Dates and times of upcoming meeting and any dates when you will *not* meet.

Opening and Closing Rituals Groups with a religious component can close each meeting quite naturally with a prayer. However, even groups that are nondenominational also benefit from opening and/or closing rituals. Many groups use a centering exercise such as deep breathing, meditation, light imagery, or affirmations.

Tip Five
Establish Ground Rules That Suit the Group's Needs

Ground rules set a disciplined tone and identify the group as being serious in its intentions. Group norms are created when you clearly state what is and what is not acceptable. If participants have the opportunity to suggest rules and decide which ones will be used, they will usually stick to them. Many groups adopt some or all of the following ground rules.

- Group always begins and ends on time.
- Confidentiality and respect for each other's privacy.
- No side conversations between group members are allowed during the meeting.
- All feelings are acceptable, whether positive or negative.
- No one monopolizes the conversation—the "10-minute rule" is followed.
- One person speaks at a time.

- Each group member is accepted without judgment.
- Sharing with others is encouraged, not required.
- Listen carefully. Give advice sparingly.

Tip Six
Provide Strong Leadership and Direction

Although your group will evolve into a self-directed community, your leadership is critically important at the first few meetings. Facilitators set the psychological climate for the group and give it direction. By creating an atmosphere of warmth, hospitality, and acceptance, you instantly provide a safe environment. When you assume a "time to work" mindset, you are letting members know that this group is important and that you intend to provide an organized agenda for each meeting—at least in the beginning. By exhibiting leadership, the facilitator minimizes anxiety because group members sense that their leaders are in control.

Tip Seven
Establish a Shared Vision/Image of the Group's Time Together

Although most people in the room know intuitively why they have come together, hearing the facilitator articulate that information clarifies the group's purpose. Prepare a brief statement describing your vision of what the group is about. Present your idea, and work with the group to redraft the vision based on their expectations of what they hope the group will accomplish.

Tip Eight
Summarize and Reflect before Closing

Each small group will develop its own personality and its own manner. A facilitator usually *senses* that personality and *feels* that tone after one or two meetings. Is this group introverted or extroverted? Hopeful or resigned? Accepting or denying? A good facilitator finds a way to verbalize that personality and tone in a positive way. At the close of each meeting, the facilitator might spend some time talking about the strengths of this particular group and how those strengths are improving with each meeting.

> By the end of our third meeting of Affirming Life, Donna and I shared with the group that we were buoyed by the fact that they had quickly developed the habit of sharing back and forth throughout the time rather than concentrating on the "group go around," a familiar pattern for most support groups. This could be for one of several reasons. First, the commonality of the women's experiences is apparent and they truly understand the feelings being expressed by others. Secondly, the size of the group (6 to 8) is the perfect size for a more intimate sharing experience.
>
> By contrast, in the larger group (15 to 20 people) that Nancy and I cofacilitate, most of the time is often spent on sharing individually, with less personal interaction. In such a group, time is limited and the environment is less intimate. Yet the group's longevity makes it feel more like a community, and just checking in on one another is sometimes enough. When serious issues arise, they support one another as needed.

FACILITATOR TIPS FOR SUBSEQUENT MEETINGS

Tip One
Be Flexible—Keep an Open Mind

There are two ways to meet difficulties: You can alter the difficulty or you can alter yourself.

—PHYLLIS BOTTOME

As early as the first or second group meeting, facilitators will probably have a good idea about the group's personality and direction. A large group will require a different structure than a very small group will. Some groups are more needy than others. Some groups tend toward the intellectual, others are more social. Some groups are simply dysfunctional. This individual makeup could mean they will quickly mesh as a group and share equally (you hope), or it could involve a mix of very withdrawn people together with one or two dominators (you hope not!).

The facilitator's challenge is to quickly size up the situation and react accordingly so that everyone in the group feels welcomed and safe—and is given an opportunity to grow. But remember, your group probably will not evolve in a way that you can predict. As the facilitator (and perhaps the person responsible for starting the group), you may have a vision of the direction *you* want the group to take. In the end, however, it's not *your* group. Go with the flow, and modify your expectations to suit the circumstances.

> *When I began facilitating my first breast cancer group, I had a vision that the members would bond quickly and then proceed to share intimate and profound insights on the challenges they faced. I thought we would get into deep, philosophical issues, as well as the fine points of human relationships. Imagine my surprise when two of our group members simply told the same story over and over again about the husband's fear of leaving the house, how the porch needed painting, or why the daughter never married.*
>
> *After two years of this, I realized the group was fulfilling a very definite purpose for these two women. I'm not certain what it is; but in terms of the group's value, that doesn't really matter. We have had other group members who have shared difficult, weighty issues, just as I expected. But today, I understand that for this group, a*

*mixture of the profound and the ordinary has become our
norm.*

Tip Two
Make Certain to Check In with Every Group
Member Each Time

If you are going to play the game properly, you'd
better know the rules.

—BARBARA JORDAN

As groups get larger and members get more comfortable with
one another, time can slip by quickly. Individual sharing
evolves into group discussion, and before you know it, it's almost closing time and you haven't heard from one or two people. Don't close without hearing from them! They may have
come to the group this time with a specific need. Allow
enough time to hear their situation. If time doesn't permit a
full discussion, ask the group to think about it and begin with
that person next time.

> *One evening, Nancy and I had a particularly large
> group. As we started around the table, I did a quick in-
> ventory and determined that John would be probably be
> our last one to speak that night. We ended up spending
> extra time on several people, and it was past 7:30 when
> we got to John. Nancy and I started to wrap it up; he had
> not jumped in with any comments, and we assumed any-
> thing could wait until next time. We were wrong. John
> had just learned that week that he was in remission from
> his lymphoma, and he had been waiting to share that
> news with the group. Although he could have broken in
> at any time, our group format dictated that he wait his
> turn in the go around. He deserved our attention, even
> though we were running late.*

Tip Three
Sprinkle Your Meetings with Humor

A person without a sense of humor is like a wagon without springs—jolted by every pebble in the road.

—Henry Ward Beecher, American clergyman

No one ever said that cancer, substance abuse, grief, death, illness, depression, battered women, or caretaking a loved one are humorous topics. Many small groups come together to support one another in times of crisis, and they will be talking about serious topics. Because of this, many group members may have been recently spending an inordinate amount of time on serious issues and could use a light break. Laughter is healthy, and the facilitator sets the stage for whether levity is acceptable in your group. Often, if the facilitator and cofacilitator joke with one another, group members will pick up on that cue and feel comfortable loosening up a bit as well.

Before I started writing the book I Can Cope: Staying Healthy with Cancer, *I needed to spend time at I Can Cope classes watching and learning from the facilitators and the class members. I can tell you I was frightened before that first class. What would it be like? Would everyone be depressed and crying? I approached with trepidation.*

Imagine my surprise when I approached the meeting room and heard laughter coming from the doorway. Wrong class? No. But the class members had learned that in the face of serious illness, a light break lifted their spirits. In our evening group, my cofacilitator Nancy brightens every meeting with self-deprecating stories of her own life—near accidents while using her cell phone in the car, or the countless difficulties of being a single-

*parent, hockey mom. Every week, she threatens deten-
tion to members who don't show up! I can't remember a
meeting going by without laughter, even when many of
our group members were seriously ill.*

*At our second Affirming Life meeting, two of our
group members realized that they were both seeing the
same doctor. One shared the story of her most recent doctor's appointment, when she brought a good friend along
as a source of support—and as a second pair of ears to listen to the doctor's advice regarding her ongoing treatment. After the visit, her friend was retelling the day's
activities to her husband, at which point she advised her
husband that "she would like that young doctor wrapped
up for a Christmas present." Sharing fun stories like this
one are a wonderful counterbalance to the tearful moments.*

Tip Four
Connect Group Members with Similar Needs

Out of suffering have emerged the strongest souls,
the most massive characters are seared with scars.

—E. J. CHAPIN

Group members with similar issues and emotions can learn
valuable coping skills from one another. Many times, these
people will gravitate toward one another without the facilitator's intervention. But an observant and intuitive facilitator
will notice similarities, whether it be age, outside interests,
type of life crisis, living arrangements, religion, age of children, and so forth. Bringing these individuals together may result in them returning to the group together. Develop a phone
list, and keep it updated to make it easier for people to contact
one another outside the group environment.

Tip Five
Follow Up Personally When Regular Members Are Absent

After the first few meetings, you will get a general sense of individuals whom you can expect to be regulars, even though open-ended groups can always expect new members. When someone misses more than one time (without letting you know in advance), a phone call is in order. Let them know they are missed—and that you are concerned about their welfare—in a way that doesn't make them feel guilty about their absence. Whatever the reason, a phone call from you signifies concern and connection.

> When Bob and his wife were missing from two consecutive meetings, Nancy followed up to find out why. After 50 plus days in the hospital being treated for leukemia just after going into remission for his prostate cancer, Bob had been an inspiration to our group as they watched him recover and become healthy once again. Now he has been in remission for two years. When Nancy called, he indicated that he felt very guilty during our meetings—he was so healthy when many of our group members were not. Nancy assured him that he remains a constant inspiration to others who strive to achieve similar success. Now he and his wife continue to come on a regular basis.

TIPS TO HELP YOU *Really* Listen

Tip #1
Focus on the Person Who Is Talking

To really concentrate on the person talking, start first by blocking all other thoughts from your own mind. Don't worry about your reaction—worry about what that person is saying.

Keep a comfortable amount of eye contact, and work hard at screening out interfering noises, words, or movements that might distract from your ability to truly hear what the person is telling you.

Tip #2
Pay Attention to What the Other Person Is Feeling

Try to walk in this person's shoes for a moment and to see the world through his or her eyes. Sometimes the words being said aren't truly indicative of the *feelings* being expressed. People may be feeling sad, or angry, or afraid, but they tell you, "I'm okay." If you respond by expressing genuine concern in saying, "You look and sound sad today," you just may reveal what is hidden beneath the surface.

Tip #3
Show That You Understand What the Person Has Said

Let the other person know that you are making a conscious effort to understand by periodically checking out what you hear. When you do this, include both the content and the feelings in what you just heard. Use short, empathetic responses. For instance, if you say, "You look and sound sad today," the speaker may, in fact, admit to feeling sad that day and tell you why. You might follow up with a statement such as: "If I'm hearing you right, it sounds to me like it's hard for you to talk about feeling sad because you don't want your family to get all concerned about you." This lets the talker know you are listening and keeps the conversation going in the right direction.

Tip #4
Try to Sort Out What Is Really Important

Some people tend to ramble from topic to topic once they get the floor. A selective listener zeros in on the relevant information, ideas, or thoughts. Then, to keep the speaker "on task," you may need to clarify the main issues. This takes some careful listening and finding an appropriate opening to provide a summary.

Tip #5
Avoid Labeling or Judging What Is Being Said

Labeling and/or evaluating often prevent you from really seeing the world through another's eyes. Rather than judging, concentrate on accepting and understanding how the person feels and how they came to hold those beliefs. Injecting your own values into this dialogue only takes the attention away from the speaker and places it back on you. Good listeners leave their own values out of the equation.

TIPS TO HELP YOU ASK GOOD QUESTIONS

Tip #1
Answer a Question with a Question

The rule might be, "Don't tell when you can ask." For instance, a common question that I get is, "Why would you want to facilitate cancer support groups? That must be depressing." Instead of instantly listing all the benefits of support groups (many of which *you* know by now), I simply say, "That's a good question. Why do you think people choose to facilitate groups?" Some people really don't understand, and they may need to be educated. But most people can figure it out if given an opportunity to think about it. This type of exploration helps group members learn more about themselves and how they think.

Tip #2
Question for Feelings as well as for Facts

If you just want to get the facts, you could ask Dennis specific questions about his life before and after AA: How many times had you been through treatment? Did the people you worked with know this was going on? How did you hide it?

But to get at the feelings, the questioning becomes more difficult: What did it feel like when you finally hit bottom? How can you describe your relationship with your sponsors? What does a higher power mean to you? Probing for feelings gets to the core of a person's motivations.

Tip #3
Avoid "Yes" or "No" Questions

Instead of asking, "Is it hard to come to the group every week?" you might ask the person, "What is hard about getting to the group every week?" By avoiding questions where people can respond with a yes or no, you are putting the ball back into their court and getting them to think about their response. By identifying reasons why coming to the group is difficult, people may begin to understand their own doubts and insecurities.

Tip #4
Return or Relay a Question Directed at You

A group member may ask you what you think about something or what you would do in a specific situation. Rather than focus on your opinions and beliefs, try to redirect the question to get the group talking. When you return the question, your response is directed at one person. For instance, if someone asks you how you feel about complementary medicine, you might say, "I'd like to know what aspect of complementary medicine interests *you.*" *Relaying a question* means throwing it back out to the group. In this case, you might say, "I'm wondering how the rest of you feel about complementary medicine."

Tips to Help You Establish Trust and to Find a Comfort Level

Tip One
To Thine Own Self Be True

> This above all: to thine own self be true,
> And it must follow, as the night the day,
> Thou canst not then be false to any man.
>
> —SHAKESPEARE, *HAMLET*

You may have attended other groups and think all groups are run the same way. Think again! Successful, ongoing groups take on a personality of their own, which is a composite of the personalities in the group. You help this process along by genuinely leading from the heart rather than by attempting to play some kind of role. Your true individual style is the *right* style. Your group is made up of individuals like yourself who have come together for a common purpose. You probably understand their reasons for attending better than anyone else, and your personal style will be appealing to them. Group members will know instinctively if you're sincere, and the only way to be sincere is to be yourself. A facilitator who can learn to relax and concentrate on the needs of the group is providing the best direction for that group.

The Guidelines for Discussion at the end of Chapters 2, 3, 4, and 5 are written to give group leaders a distinct format and template for some specific group discussions. But they are not all-inclusive, and they don't take into account the variables among presenters and groups. A successful facilitator knows what feels most comfortable and will adapt to the direction the group is taking. For instance, the two Discussion Guides at the end of Chapter 2 (Getting to Know One Another and Discovering the Power of Words) are designed for groups that are just forming.

Tip Two
Get Personal with Your Group

Just be what you are and speak from your guts and heart—it's all a man has.

—HUBERT H. HUMPHREY

At the first meeting, you might tell a personal story that clarifies why you were committed to initiating (or joining in with) this group. Because your story is extremely meaningful to *you*, it was probably a strong motivator for your actions. The sincerity with which you tell your story will come through loud and clear and will help connect you with other group members. Personal disclosures serve as powerful ice breakers, instantly forging a bond between the facilitator and other group members. I told you my personal story at the very beginning of this book to help you understand more about me and why support groups are important to me. As a follow-up to that story, my mother was diagnosed with breast cancer at the age of 80 and died of Alzheimer's disease at the age of 89. My oldest sister was diagnosed with breast cancer at the age of 60. For this day, I am still healthy.

GROUP LEADER'S SKILLS SUMMARY

You are helping when you—

- Listen with your full attention.
- Are organized and prepared before the beginning of each meeting.
- Participate by *encouraging*, not *directing*.
- Structure meetings early in the group's formation.
- Use humor to reduce distress or to bring people together.

- Disclose information about yourself to draw out the feelings of others.
- Provide information without lecturing.
- Accept each person's position without judging them.
- Identify common group themes.
- Ask questions in specific ways so the group is guided in the proper direction.
- Put people's feelings and behavior into words the group can understand.
- Protect members from verbally injuring one another.
- Encourage everyone to talk without pressuring anyone.
- Invite silent members to participate.
- Communicate nonverbally by using eye contact, body language, and nodding of your head.
- Exhibit a caring attitude by displaying warmth and affection to group members.
- Cope with conflict when it arises instead of ignoring it.
- Encourage individuals to take ownership in the group by assigning tasks.
- Connect individuals with one another based on mutual needs and experiences.
- Summarize the group's progress and learnings at the conclusion of each meeting.
- Refer individuals needing special help to the appropriate source.

You are not *helping when you—*

- Take over the discussion or start to lecture.
- Are confrontational or argumentative.
- Suggest solutions rather than listening without passing judgment.
- Minimize the importance of feelings being expressed.
- Withhold warmth and affection.
- Allow any disruptive behavior to continue and form a pattern.
- Avoid discussion of tough issues.

FACILITATOR TIPS FOR CHALLENGING SITUATIONS

The following are sample statements that you might use when difficult situations arise.

When a group member has been upstaged without completing his or her sharing time—

- I'm concerned that we've taken the conversation away from _____. I'd like to get back to him/her before we move on.
- I'm concerned about _____.

When a group member is having trouble getting to the point or is rambling in an unclear manner—

- I'm confused. Could someone help me understand what just happened here?
- Can you say how this situation is affecting you now?
- Could anyone respond by talking about a similar situation you have had?

When a group member seems uncertain of their direction or of their decisions—

- You seem to be encouraged by the progress you've made so far. Will you keep going in this same direction?
- Is that what *you* want?
- What choices do you think you have in this situation?

When a group member jumps from topic to topic with no clear direction—

- Of the several things you have mentioned, is there one thing you would like us to focus on right now?

- Can another group member respond to any of these topics by relating them to a similar situation in your life?

When the meeting time is running short and closure is near—

- Is there any unfinished business we need to deal with before we end?

SUPPORT GROUPS
WHY DO PEOPLE JOIN—
AND WHY DO THEY STAY?

People join support groups to:

- Share common experiences and problems.
- Talk and/or listen.
- Share in problem solving and offer solutions.
- Have an emotional outlet and to gain support from peers.
- Reduce isolation.
- Find a sense of community.
- Form new friendships.
- Learn self-help techniques.
- Develop new skills through education and advocacy.
- Help others while helping self.

People stop attending groups because:

- They didn't feel welcome or accepted.
- The group didn't meet their individual needs.
- They felt pressured, embarrassed, or confused.
- The group had a negative focus.
- Friends stopped attending.
- They had gotten all the help they wanted and no longer felt the need.
- They weren't involved or committed.

- The group became stagnant and didn't foster new growth.
- The group lacked leadership or direction.

People don't join support groups because they:

- Don't view them as a personal necessity—don't sense the need.
- Don't know anything about the group and are wary.
- Feel uncomfortable talking about themselves in front of others.
- Lack transportation.
- Don't want to go alone.

MUTUAL-HELP GROUPS FOSTERING NEW GROWTH

One of the greatest challenges faced by group organizers is keeping the group active and interested. People want to believe that they are making a difference and that the group is making a difference in their lives. The following suggestions may help group leaders maintain a membership base while still attracting new members.

- *Develop a mentor system.* When new members join the group, try to match them with a veteran group member in a similar situation. The veteran member helps the new member learn the ropes of exactly how your group operates. This makes the new person feel welcome, and it gives the veteran member a sense of responsibility and ownership in the group process.
- *Regularly reassess the group's needs.* As groups grow and mature, they may develop a different focus. Group leaders should be querying the group regularly to get a feel for their current needs and to plan the focus topics accordingly.

- *Help members assume ownership.* When members assume some form of ownership, they are more likely to stay. Think creatively about assigning task responsibilities to members; for example, someone could be given the task of coordinating refreshments. Individual tasks assign meaning and make individual members relevant to the group's success.

SAMPLE PUBLIC SERVICE ANNOUNCEMENT (PSA)

(For use on radio and television)

Public Service Announcement
(Date)

Contact: _____(facilitator's name)_____
                        _____(address)_____
                        _____(phone)_____

For Immediate Release

(30 seconds)

If you—or someone in your family—has recently (define the life crisis), you may feel like you are the only one trying to understand the immense changes in your life. Be assured that others have similar feelings. And now there's a safe place to share those feelings. A newly formed support group meets regularly to help people understand the changes brought on by _____. The group members help one another understand those changes and offer coping mechanisms for change. They meet on (enter meeting date) at (enter meeting time) at (enter meeting location). If you want more information about the group, call (enter facilitator's name and telephone number).

SAMPLE PRESS RELEASE

(For any newspaper or print media)

For Immediate Release

Contact:
Phone:
E-Mail

Begin Date
End Date

If you, someone in your family, or a friend has been affected by (name the life crisis or situation), a unique support program is being organized in your community. At each meeting, group members learn more about _____ by sharing their own experiences. Together, they help one another understand coping strategies for the future. The goal of the support program is to provide encouragement and guidance and to help individuals learn adaptive skills that will assist them in learning to live with a changed life. The first meeting will be held on (meeting date) at (meeting time) at (exact meeting location, including room number, if possible). All interested persons are encouraged to attend.

SAMPLE GROUND RULES

- We are a group of people with a common bond, sharing our concerns, feelings, experiences, strength, and wisdom.
- We listen with understanding, but we don't judge or offer solutions.
- We operate as a group, and we don't tolerate side conversations.
- We have equal opportunity to be heard and can share as much—or as little—as we wish.
- We don't interrupt when someone else is talking.
- We encourage "I" statements and speak only from our own experience.
- We avoid giving medical advice or mentioning the names of health providers or medical institutions.
- We share responsibility in making the group successful.
- We take turns in all things, including speaking, listening, and group leadership, so that no one person can become a monopolizer.
- We accept all members and their feelings without judging.

Suggested Reading

The following books have helped me either in my research for writing this book or in my capacity as a group leader. I hope you will find them enjoyable as well.

A Circle of Men by Bill Kauth. New York: St. Martin's Press, 1992.

This book gives wonderful practical suggestions for men who want to start a group specifically for men. Not only does the author have personal experience, but he provides a great deal of information on topics for discussion, a great book list for men, and many structured learning activities.

Healing and the Mind by Bill Moyers. New York: Doubleday, 1993.

This timeless book includes interviews with a variety of health care professionals on topics such as the art of healing, the mind/body connection, and the interconnectedness of life and death. The insights uncovered in the interviews provide a well-balanced look at the healing process.

The Healing Power of Humor by Allen Klein. New York: Jeremy P. Tarcher/Putnam, 1989.

This is a delightful and informational book regarding the value of humor to help you get through loss, setbacks, upsets, difficulties, and so forth. Klein has a good medical understanding of what makes people sick— and he provides practical ways to use humor when faced with a variety of difficult situations.

Health Online: How to Find Health Information, Support Groups, and Self-Help Communities in Cyberspace by Tom Ferguson. Reading, MA: Addison-Wesley, 1996.

This book makes going online easy by explaining e-mail and by showing what's on the big commercial online services. He explores Internet mailing lists, newsgroups, and World Wide Web pages. He also lists hundreds of self-help support groups. An excellent resource for individuals seeking support in cyberspace.

I Can Cope: Staying Healthy with Cancer by Judi Johnson and Linda Klein. Minneapolis, MN: Chronimed, 1994.

This book was written to coincide with the American Cancer Society's educational program for people with cancer and their families. The information is easy to understand and covers a variety of issues surrounding a cancer diagnosis. In particular, chapters on support systems, communication, and staying healthy are useful for anyone facing a chronic condition.

Kitchen Table Wisdom by Rachel Naomi Remen, M.D. New York: Riverhead Books, 1994.

I like to read excerpts from this book as the closing ritual for every support group meeting. Dr. Remen is a pediatrician by training and has served as the Medical Director of the Commonweal Cancer Help Program. She has worked closely with the small-group process and has observed the interaction among people in crisis. Her insights into human nature and the sanctity of human connection are realistic and moving.

Living beyond Limits: New Hope and Help for Facing Life-Threatening Illness by David Spiegel, M.D. New York: Random House, 1993.

Spiegel's book draws on his support group experience as he was conducting research to determine the value of a supportive environment for women with metastatic breast cancer. His amazing results showed that the women in the support group lived 18 months longer than the control group. This book gives excellent information on what happens in a supportive group and why it is valuable.

Manifesto for a New Medicine by Jim Gordon, M.D. Reading, MA: Addison-Wesley, 1996.

Dr. Gordon is a Harvard-trained physician who went on to develop the Center for Mind-Body Medicine in Washington, D.C. He is an innovative thinker and a true believer in the mind/body approach to health and healing.

No Time for Nonsense: Self Help for the Seriously Ill by Ronna Fay Jevne, Ph.D., and Alexander Levitan, M.D. San Diego, CA: Luramedia, 1989.

Much like the book *The Healing Power of Humor,* this book is a practical guide for looking at the bright side of a serious condition. It talks about stress, gaining perspective, anger, depression, support systems, and many other important relationship-oriented issues.

Sharing the Journey: Support Groups and America's New Quest for Community by Robert Wuthnow. New York: Free Press, 1994.

Wuthnow's book takes a very close look at the small-group movement, particularly church-related groups dealing with marital, parenting, youth, spiritual, and other problem issues. As a sociologist at Princeton University, he has done considerable research on small groups, and his findings suggest that a "quiet revolution" is taking place in the United States as more and more people are finding satisfaction within the small-group environment.

Support Group Leader's Guide by Jennie Newbrough. Lynnwood, WA: Women's Aglow Fellowship, 1993.

This book wouldn't be for everyone, but it will be helpful for a Christian who is interested in starting a church-focused group. The author has good insight into group development, and she augments her writing with passages from scripture.

Additional Resources
for Finding Support Nationwide

American Association of Retired People (AARP)
601 E Street, NW
Washington, DC 20049
(800) 424-3410, (202) 434-2277
www.aarp.org

AARP provides a wide range of services to people aged 50 or over. Services include information, counseling groups, advocacy, benefits and entitlement, community activities, employment opportunities, teaching opportunities, training, and assistance to the homebound. A bimonthly magazine is available.

American Brain Tumor Association (ABTA)
2720 River Road, Suite 146
Des Plaines, IL 60018
(800) 886-2282, (847) 827-9910, FAX (847) 827-9918
www.abta.org
E-mail: info@abta.org

This national organization provides patients and family members with written information about brain tumors and treatment. Services include patient education materials, a listing of support groups, referrals to support organizations, a pen-pal program, information on treatment facilities, and funding for research. ABTA also publishes a newsletter and provides publications for the public.

American Foundation for Urologic Disease
1128 North Charles Street
Baltimore, MD 21201
0)468-1800, FAX (410) 468-1808
www.afud.org
   Provides information on support groups for prostate cancer survivors and their families, as well as information on prostate cancer and other urologic disorders. A national information/referral service, including a phone line, is available.

American Self-Help Clearinghouse
St. Clare's Health Services
25 Pocono Road
Denville, NJ 07834
(973) 625-3037, (973) 625-9053
www.cmhc.com/selfhelp
   The American Self-Help Clearinghouse puts callers in touch with any of several hundred national and international self-help groups covering a wide range of illnesses, disabilities, addictions, bereavement, and stressful life situations. It has compiled a national database of over 800 of these and model groups. They also provide referrals to local self-help clearinghouses that exist in some states. The Clearinghouse provides information and consultation nationally to help people start new types of self-help groups when none currently exist. They publish a national directory and a Network newsletter containing articles of interest to the self-help and professional community. Assistance for people interested in starting support groups is provided by telephone consultation and with resource materials by mail.

Bone Marrow Transplant Family Support Network
PO Box 845
Avon, CT 06001
(800) 826-9376

This national person-to-person support network enables families to feel connected when coping with the transplant decision, with daily routines prior to and following transplants, and with the follow-up care after transplant.

Cancer Care, Inc.
275 7th Avenue
New York, NY 10001
(212) 221-3300 (national office), (800) 813-HOPE (813-4673)
www.cancercare.org
E-mail: info@cancercare.org

Cancer Care is a nonprofit organization whose mission is to help people with cancer and their families. Through professional one-to-one counseling, support groups, educational programs, and telephone contact, Cancer Care provides guidance, information, and referrals to cancer patients and families, all free of charge. Cancer Care also offers limited financial assistance for treatment-related costs on a restricted basis in New York City, Long Island, New Jersey, and Connecticut. Cancer Care provides direct services through offices in New York, New Jersey, and Connecticut and nationally through their toll-free number.

Cancer Support Network
Essex House, Suite L10
Baum Boulevard at South Negley Avenue
Pittsburgh, PA 15206
(412) 361-8600

This is a professional and peer-support network for cancer survivors, family, and friends.

Candlelighters Childhood Cancer Foundation
7910 Woodmont Avenue, Suite 460
Bethesda, MD 20814-3015
(800)366-2223, (301) 657-8401
www.candlelighters.org
E-mail: info@candlelighters.org
   The Foundation provides support, information, and advocacy regarding childhood cancer and referral to local self-help groups. CCCF has a network of peer support groups for parents; publishes a Quarterly Newsletter, Youth Newsletter, bibliography, and other materials; answers information requests; and maintains an Ombudsman Program on insurance concerns and long-term survivors' network. Other services include bereavement counseling, pain management, speaker's bureau, and a phone line.

CHEMOcare
231 North Avenue, West
Westfield, NJ 07090
(800) 55-CHEMO (552-4366), (908) 233-1103 (NJ residents)
   This program of personal support and encouragement is offered to people undergoing chemotherapy and/or radiation therapy by people who have experienced the treatment themselves. Other services include a newsletter, volunteer training programs, cancer counseling, self-help/peer support groups, family and individual groups, cancer information, patient advocacy, speaker's bureau, information/referrals for community resources, and a phone line.

The Compassionate Friends
P.O. Box 3696
Oak Brook, Illinois 60522-3696
(630) 990-0010, FAX (630) 990-0246
www.compassionatefriends.org
   The mission of The Compassionate Friends is to assist families in the positive resolution of grief following the death

of a child and to provide information to help others be supportive.

Encore Plus
Bess Chisum Stephens YWCA
1200 Cleveland Street
Little Rock, AR 72204
(501) 663-8111, FAX (501) 663-0204
www.ywcaencore.org
E-mail: healthhelp@ywcaencore.org
   Encore Plus targets medically underserved women over 50 in need of early detection education, breast and cervical cancer screening, and support services. It offers a unique combined peer-support-and-exercise program for women receiving treatment and/or recovering from breast cancer.

The Humor Project
480 Broadway, Suite 210
Saratoga Springs, NY 12866-2288
(518) 587-8770, FAX (518) 587-8771
www.humorproject.com
E-mail: questions@HumorProject.com
   It provides a free catalog and resources on humorous material, and it holds conferences on the use of humor in coping with illness.

Let's Face It
Box 711
Concord, MA 01742
(508) 371-3186
   This is a mutual-help network for the facially disfigured.

Leukemia Society of America
600 Third Avenue
New York, NY 10016
(800) 955-4LSA, (212) 573-8484
www.leukemia.org

This agency is dedicated to finding causes and cures for leukemia, lymphomas (including Hodgkin's disease), and multiple myeloma. All counseling groups are free of charge and open to patients and families. Other services available are financial assistance, funding grants, professional education, speaker bureau, publications, literature, and information/referrals to different resources.

Make Today Count
c/o Connie Zimmerman
Mid-America Cancer Center
1235 East Cherokee
Springfield, MO 65804-2263
(800) 432-2273, FAX (417) 888-7426

This mutual-support organization brings together people affected by a life-threatening illness so they may help each other. More than 200 chapters in the United States provide formal programs, group discussions, chapter newsletters, social activities, workshops and seminars, and education activities.

National Alliance of Breast Cancer Organizations (NABCO)
9 East 37th Street, 10th Floor
New York, NY 10016
(212) 719-0154, (800) 719-9154 (outside New York City),
(212) 889-0606
www.nabco.org
E-mail: info@nabco.org

NABCO, established in 1986, is a nonprofit central resource for information and education about breast cancer, with a network of more than 375 organizations that provide detection, treatment, and care to American women. In addition to disseminating information, NABCO advocates for regulatory change and legislation that benefits breast cancer patients, survivors, and women at risk. Other services include job-discrimination-related issues, professional education, speaker's bureau, and literature/publications for the public.

National Brain Tumor Foundation (NBTF)
785 Market Street, Suite 1600
San Francisco, CA 94103
(800) 934-CURE, (415) 284-0208
www.braintumor.org
E-mail: nbtf@braintumor.org

This Foundation raises funds for research and provides information on local and national levels. It also offers counseling/support services to brain tumor patients, survivors, and their families. Issues a quarterly newsletter. A telephone support line also is available for patient-to-patient contact. An excellent publication, "Brain Tumors: The Resource Guide," is available free of charge.

National Coalition for Cancer Survivorship (NCCS)
1010 Wayne Avenue, 5th Floor
Silver Spring, MD 20910
(301) 650-8868, FAX (301) 565-9670

NCCS is a network of independent groups and individuals concerned with survivorship and support of cancer survivors and their loved ones. The primary goal is to promote national awareness of issues affecting cancer survivors. The NCCS serves as a clearinghouse for information on services and for materials on survivorship; encourages the study of survivorship; and promotes the development of cancer support activities.

National Domestic Violence Hotline
1-800-799-SAFE (7233), 1-800-787-3224 (TTY)
www.ndvh.org

Each month, nearly 10,000 callers—victims of domestic violence, their families, and their friends across the United States—receive crisis intervention, referrals, information, and support in many languages. One call summons immediate help, in English or Spanish, 24 hours a day, 7 days a week. The Hotline links individuals to help in their area using a nationwide database that includes detailed information on domestic violence shelters, other emergency shelters, legal advocacy and assistance programs, and social service programs.

National Family Caregivers Association
9621 East Bexhill Drive
Kensington, MD 20895
(800) 896-3650, (301) 942-6430
It helps improve lives of America's 18 million caregivers by providing information and support.

National Hospice Organization
1901 North Moore Street, Suite 901
Arlington, VA 22209
Referrals (800) 658-8898, office (703) 243-5900
www.nho.org
E-mail: drshho@cais.com
This nonprofit membership association is dedicated to promoting and maintaining quality care of terminally ill people and their families and to providing education, technical assistance, publications, and advocacy and referral services.

National Infertility Network Exchange
PO Box 204
East Meadow, NY 11554
(516) 794-5772
This clearinghouse provides information on peer support groups for infertile couples, education programs, and has a referral service.

National Lymphedema Network
2211 Post Street, Suite 404
San Francisco, CA 94115
(800) 541-3259, FAX (415) 921-4284
www.lymphnet.org
This nonprofit resource center provides information about prevention and treatment of lymphedema, swelling that is a

common complication of lymph node surgery. They help organize local support groups focusing on the treatment and impact of lymphedema and publish a newsletter with personal stories as well as network news.

National Resource Center for Family Support Programs
Family Resource Coalition
200 North Wacker Drive, Suite 1100
Chicago, IL 60606
(312) 338-0900
www.frca.org
    This group publishes a 23-page guide, *Starting and Operating Support Groups,* including suggestions, flyers, meeting handouts, resource directory, and a guide for finding parenting support resources in the community.

National Self-Help Clearinghouse
CUNY, Graduate School and University Center
25 West 43rd Street, Room 620
New York, NY 10036
(212) 642-2944, FAX (212) 642-1956
www.selfhelpweb.org
    The National Self-Help Clearinghouse collects and distributes information about self-care and self-help groups throughout the country and provides technical assistance and advice to these groups. The Clearinghouse serves as an information-and-referral service, providing information to the public about self-help groups, helping networks, and community support systems. It also offers training programs to self-help group leaders and publishes manuals, training materials, and a newsletter.

Prostate Cancer Support Group Network
300 West Pratt Street, Suite 401
Baltimore, MD 21201
(410) 727-2908

A national network of over 400 prostate cancer survivor support and self-help groups that promotes awareness, education, support, and research. The network addresses the collective needs of all the groups through increasing public awareness and advocacy and provides current information through leadership meetings and educational seminars.

SHARE
St. Joseph Health Center
300 First Capitol Drive
St. Charles, MO 63301-2893
(800) 821-6819, (636) 947-6164, FAX (636) 947-7486
www.nationalshareoffice.com
SHARE serves those whose lives are touched by the tragic death of a baby. The purpose is to provide support toward positive resolution of grief and to provide education and support regarding resources for bereaved parents and siblings.

US TOO International, Inc.
930 North York Road, Suite 50
Hinsdale, IL 60521-2993
(800) 808-7866, (630) 323-1002, FAX (630) 323-1003
www.ustoo.com
US TOO is an independent network of support group chapters for men with prostate cancer and their families. US TOO groups offer fellowship, peer counseling, education about treatment options, and discussion of medical alternatives without bias.

Wellness Community
2716 Ocean Park Boulevard, Suite 1040
Santa Monica, CA 90405-5211
(310) 314-2555
The Wellness Community is the largest cancer support organization devoted solely to psychological and emotional support for cancer survivors and their families. The organization

serves as an adjunct to medical treatment. All services are free, including support groups, workshops, lectures, and other social events.

Well Spouse Foundation
30 East 40th Street, PH
New York, NY 10018
(212) 685-8815, (800) 838-0879, FAX (212) 685-8676
www.wellspouse.org

The Well Spouse Foundation is a national, not-for-profit membership organization that gives support to husbands, wives, and partners of people with chronic illness and/or disabilities. It provides a bimonthly newsletter, mutual-aid support groups in many areas, letter-writing support groups, and an annual conference. The organization also works with health care professionals and the general public to increase awareness of the great difficulties that caregivers face every day.

Bibliography

Barnes, R. "Problems of families caring for Alzheimer's patients: Use of a support group." *Journal of the American Geriatric Society* 24, 2 (1981) 80–85.

Bormann, Ernest G., and Nancy C. Bormann. *Effective Small Group Communication.* Minneapolis, MN: Burgess Publishing, 1988.

Bruhn, John G., and Stewart Wolf. *The Roseto Story: An Anatomy of Health.* New York: Harper and Row, 1979.

Burnside, Irene, and Mary Gwynne Schmidt. *Working with Older Adults.* London: Jones and Bartlett, 1994.

Bruner, Jerome. "Life as Narrative." *Social Research* 54 (1987), 12.

Caplan, G., and Killelea M. Caplan. *Support Systems and Mutual Help.* New York: Grune & Stratton, 1976.

Caserta, M. S., and D. A. Lund. "Intrapersonal Resources and the Effectiveness of Self-Help Groups for Bereaved Older Adults." *Gerontologist* 33, no. 5 (1993) 619–629.

Cella, David F., and Suzanne B. Yellen. "Cancer support groups: The state of the art." *Cancer Practice* 1, 1 (1993), 56–61.

De Becker, Gavin. "Why I Fight Abuse." *USA Weekend*, May 14–16, 1999, p. 14.

DeToqueville, Alexis. *Democracy in America,* 2 vols. New York: Vantage, 1945.

Dossey, Larry, M.D. *Healing Words: The Power of Prayer and the Practice of Medicine*. San Francisco: HarperCollins, 1993.

Edmunson, E. D., J. R. Bedell, et al. "Integrating Skill Building and Peer Support in Mental Health Treatment: The Early Intervention and Community Network Development Projects." In *Community Mental Health and Behavioral Ecology*, edited by A. M. Jeger and R. S. Slotnick, 127–139. New York: Plenum Press, 1982.

Emrick, C. D., J. S. Tonigan, et al. "Alcoholics Anonymous: What Is Currently Known?" In *Research on Alcoholics Anonymous: Opportunities and Alternatives*, edited by Barbara S. McCrady and William R. Miller, 41–75. New Brunswick, NJ: Rutgers Center of Alcohol Studies, 1993.

Frankl, Viktor E. *Man's Search for Meaning*. New York: Washington Square Press, Simon & Schuster, 1963.

Gilden, J. L., M. S. Hendryx, et al. "Diabetes Support Groups Improve Health Care of Older Diabetic Patients." *Journal of the American Geriatrics Society* 40 (1992) 147–150.

Gordon, James S., M.D. *Manifesto for a New Medicine: Your Guide to Healing Partnerships and the Wise Use of Alternative Therapies*. Reading, MA: Addison Wesley, 1996.

Guidelines on Support and Self-Help Groups. Atlanta, GA: American Cancer Society, 1992.

Heider, J. *The Tao of Leadership*. New York: Bantam Books, 1985.

Hill, K. *Helping You Helps Me: A Guide for Self-Help Groups*. Ottawa, Ontario: Canadian Council on Social Development, 1984.

Hoffman, Barbara, ed. *A Cancer Survivor's Almanac—Charting Your Journey*. Minnetonka, MN: Chronimed Publishing, 1996.

Hughes, J. M. "Adolescent Children of Alcoholic Parents and the Relationship of Alateen to These Children." *Journal of Consulting and Clinical Psychology* 45, no. 5 (1977) 946–947.

I Can Cope Facilitator's Guide. Atlanta, GA: American Cancer Society, 1994.

Jason, L. A., C. L. Gruder, et al. "Work Site Group Meetings and the Effectiveness of a Televised Smoking Cessation Intervention." *American Journal of Community Psychology* 15 (1987) 57–77.

Jevne, Ronna Fay, and Alexander Levitan. *No Time for Nonsense: Self-Help for the Seriously Ill.* San Diego, CA: Lura-Media, 1989.

Johnson, David. *Reaching Out.* Englewood Cliffs, NJ: Prentice Hall, 1972.

Johnson, George, David Mayer, and Nancy Vogel. *Starting Small Groups and Keeping Them Going.* Minneapolis, MN: Augsburg Fortress Press, 1995.

Johnson, Judi, and Linda Klein. *I Can Cope: Staying Healthy with Cancer.* Minnetonka, MN: Chronimed Publishing, 1994.

Johnson, Judi, and C. Lane. "Role of support groups in cancer care." *Supportive Care in Cancer* 1 (1993) 52–56.

Katz, A., and E. Bender. "Self-help groups in Western society: history and prospects." *Journal of Applied Behavioral Sciences* 12 (1976) 265–282.

Kauth, Bill. *A Circle of Men: The Original Manual for Men's Support Groups.* New York: St. Martin's Press, 1992.

Kennedy, M. "Psychiatric Hospitalizations of GROWers." Paper presented at the Second Biennial Conference on Comity Research and Action, East Lansing, MI, 1990.

Kirschenbaum, Howard, and Barbara Glaser. *Developing Support Groups: A Manual for Facilitators and Participants.* La Jolla, CA: University Associates, 1978.

Klein, Allen. *The Healing Power of Humor.* New York: Putnam, Jeremy P. Tarcher/Perigree, 1989.

Klein, Linda L., and Judi Johnson. *Discovery Circles,* National Stroke Association's Guide to Organizing and Facilitating Stroke Support Groups, 1997. Denver, CO: NSA.

Kurtz, L. F. "Mutual Aid for Affective Disorders: The Manic Depressive and Depressive Association," *American Journal of Orthopsychiatry* 58, no. 1 (1988) 152–155.

Lerner, Michael. *Choices in Healing: Integrating the Best of Conventional and Complementary Approaches to Cancer.* Cambridge, MA: MIT Press, 1996.

Marshall, J. R., and D. P. Funch. "Social Environment and Breast Cancer: A Cohort Analysis of Breast Cancer." *Cancer* 52 (1983) 1546–1550.

Mayer, Musa. *Holding Tight, Letting Go: Living wth Metastatic Breast Cancer.* Sebastopol, CA: O'Reilly and Associates, 1997.

Mitchell, W. J. T., ed. *On Narrative.* Chicago: University of Chicago Press, 1981.

Moyers, Bill. *Healing and the Mind.* New York: Doubleday, 1993.

Newbrough, Jennie, with Carol Greenwood. *Support Group Leader's Guide.* Lynnwood, WA: *Women's Aglow Fellowship International,* 1993.

Ornish, Dean. *Dr. Dean Ornish's Program for Reversing Heart Disease.* New York: Random House, 1990.

Ornstein, Robert, and David Sobel. *The Healing Brain: Breakthrough Discoveries about How the Brain Keeps Us Healthy.* New York: Simon & Schuster, 1987.

Pierce, Linda L., and Judith P. Salter. "Stroke support group: A reality." *Rehabilitation Nursing* 13, no. 4 (1988) 189–190, 197.

Redwood, Daniel. *Interviews with People Who Make a Difference.* Larry Dossey, 1995.

Remen, Rachel Naomi, M.D. *Kitchen Table Wisdom.* New York: Riverhead Books, 1994.

Ryan, Cornelius, and Katherine Ryan Morgan. *A Private Battle.* New York: Simon & Schuster, 1979.

Sampson, Edward E. *Group Process for the Health Professional.* New York: Delmar, 1990.

Schiff, Harriot Sarnoff. *The Support Group Manual.* New York: Penguin Books, 1996.

Self-Help: What Is It? www.selfhelpweb.org [cited July 27, 1998].

Shaffer, Carolyn R., and Kristin Anundsen. *Creating Community Anywhere: Finding Support and Connection in a Fragmented World.* New York: Putnam, Jeremy P. Tarcher/ Penguin, 1993.

Smith, Donna Rae. *The Power of Building Your Bright Side.* Grand Rapids, MI: Baker Book House, Wynwood, 1995.

The Social Seminar Facilitator Material. Washington, D.C.: National Institute of Mental Health. Government Printing Office, 1971.

Spiegel, David, M.D. *Living Beyond Limits: New Hope and Help for Facing Life-Threatening Illness.* New York: Random House, 1993.

Spiegel, David, M.D. "A Psychosocial Intervention and Survival Time of Patients with Metastatic Breast Cancer," *Advances 7,* 3 (Summer 1991) 10–19.

Spiegel, David, J. Bloom, H. C. Kraemer, and E. Gottheil. "The Effect of Psychosocial Treatment on Survival of Metastatic Breast Cancer Patients: A Randomized Prospective Outcome Study." *The Lancet* (October 14, 1989) 888–891.

Spiegel, D., J. Bloom, and I. Yalom. "Group Support for Patients with Metastatic Cancer." *Archives of General Psychiatry* 38 (1981) 527–533.

Toseland, R. W., C. M. Rossiter, and M. S. Labrecque. "The Effectiveness of Two Kinds of Support Groups for Caregivers." *Social Service Review,* September (1989) 415–432.

Videka-Sherman, L., and M. Lieberman. "The Effects of Self-Help and Psychotherapy Intervention on Child Loss: The Limits of Recovery." *American Journal of Orthopsychiatry* 55, no. 1 (1985) 70–82.

Vugia, H. D. "Support groups in oncology: Building hope through the human bond." *Journal of Psychosocial Oncology* 9, 3 (1991) 89–107.

Wasserman, Harry, and H. E. Danforth. *The Human Bond: Support Groups and Mutual Aid.* New York: Springer, 1988.

Wuthnow, Robert. *Sharing the Journey: Support Groups and America's New Quest for Community.* New York: Simon & Schuster, Free Press, 1994.

Yalom, Irvin D. *Existential Psychotherapy.* New York: Basic Books, 1980.

Index